KV-195-971

PREVENTION AND TREATMENT OF OSTEOPOROSIS: A CLINICIAN'S GUIDE

Edited by

Cyrus Cooper MA DM FRCP

MRC Environmental Epidemiology Unit,
Southampton General Hospital,
Tremona Road, Southampton
SO16 6YD, UK

Stephen Gehlbach MD MPH

School of Public Health and Health Sciences,
University of Massachusetts at Amherst,
MA 01003, USA

Robert Lindsay MD PhD

Department of Internal Medicine,
Helen Hayes Hospital, West Haverstraw,
NY 10993 and Columbia University NY, USA

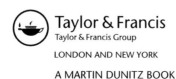

Taylor & Francis
Taylor & Francis Group
LONDON AND NEW YORK

A MARTIN DUNITZ BOOK

© 2005 Taylor & Francis, an imprint of the Taylor & Francis Group

First published in the United Kingdom in 2005
by Taylor & Francis, an imprint of the Taylor & Francis Group, 2 Park Square, Milton Park,
Abingdon, Oxfordshire, OX14 4RN.

Tel.:   +44 (0) 20 7017 6000
Fax.:   +44 (0) 20 7017 6699
E-mail: info@dunitz.co.uk
Website: http://www.dunitz.co.uk

All rights reserved. No part of this publication may be reproduced, stored in a retrieval
system, or transmitted, in any form or by any means, electronic, mechanical, photocopying,
recording, or otherwise, without the prior permission of the publisher or in accordance with
the provisions of the Copyright, Designs and Patents Act 1988 or under the terms of any
licence permitting limited copying issued by the Copyright Licensing Agency, 90 Tottenham
Court Road, London W1P 0LP.

Although every effort has been made to ensure that all owners of copyright material have
been acknowledged in this publication, we would be glad to acknowledge in subsequent
reprints or editions any omissions brought to our attention.

A CIP record for this book is available from the British Library.

Library of Congress Cataloging-in-Publication Data

Data available on application

ISBN 1 84184 283 4

Distributed in North and South America by

Taylor & Francis
2000 NW Corporate Blvd
Boca Raton, FL 33431, USA

Within Continental USA
Tel: 800 272 7737; Fax: 800 374 3401
Outside Continental USA
Tel: 561 994 0555; Fax: 561 361 6018
E-mail: orders@crcpress.com

Distributed in the rest of the world by
Thomson Publishing Services
Cheriton House
North Way
Andover, Hampshire SP10 5BE, UK
Tel.: +44 (0)1264 332424
E-mail: salesorder.tandf@thomsonpublishingservices.co.uk

Composition J&L Composition, Filey, North Yorkshire, UK
Printed and bound in Great Britain by Cromwell Press Ltd

Contents

Contributors v

1 Perspectives on the problem 1
  Cyrus Cooper and Stephen Gehlbach

2 Epidemiology 13
  L Joseph Melton, III

3 Pathophysiology of osteoporosis 27
  Cyrus Cooper

4 Risk stratification 43
  John A Kanis

5 The treatment of postmenopausal osteoporosis 57
  Pierre D Delmas

6 Economic aspects of osteoporosis 81
  Rachael L Fleurence, Cynthia P Iglesias and David J Torgerson

7 Strategies for prevention 103
  Stephen Gehlbach

Index 119

STEPPING HILL HOSPITAL
LIBRARY
PINEWOOD HOUSE

Contributors

Cyrus Cooper MA DM FRCP
Professor of Rheumatology
MRC Environmental Epidemiology Unit
Southampton General Hospital
Tremona Road
Southampton SO16 6YD
UK

Pierre D Delmas MD PhD
Professor of Medicine
Hôpital Edouard Herriot
Pavillon F
69437 Lyon Cedex 03
France

Rachel L Fleurence
MRC Phd Student
Seebohm Rowntree Building (Area 4)
York Trials Unit
Department of Health Sciences & Centre for Health Economics
University of York
York YO10 5DD
UK

Stephen Gehlbach MD MPH
Professor
School of Public Health and Health Sciences
University of Massachusetts at Amherst
Amherst, MA 01003
USA

Cynthia P Iglesias
Research Fellow
Seebohm Rowntree Building (Area 2)
Department of Health Sciences & Centre for Health Economics
University of York
York YO10 5DD
UK

John A Kanis MD FRCP FRCPath
Professor
WHO Collaborating Centre for Metabolic Diseases
University of Sheffield Medical School
Beech Hill Road
Sheffield S10 2RX
UK

Robert Lindsay Chief MD PhD
Professor of Clinical Medicine
Columbia University, NY, and
Chief
Department of Internal Medicine
Helen Hayes Hospital
West Haverstraw, NY 10993
USA

L Joseph Melton III MD
Professor of Epidemiology
Department of Health Sciences Research
Mayo Medical School
200 First Street SW
Rochester, MN 55905
USA

David J Torgerson PhD
Professor of Health Economics
Department of Health Sciences & Centre for Health Economics
University of York
York YO10 5DD
UK

1

Perspectives on the problem

Cyrus Cooper and Stephen Gehlbach

The concept of a condition in which physiologically weakened bone contributes to excessive fractures has developed over the past 180 years. The earliest description in the English literature of osteoporotic fracture and identification of factors that place an individual at high risk for the condition appeared in the early 1820s.[1] Sir Astley Cooper noted that the London hospital wards of Guys' and St Thomas' were 'seldom without an example of fracture of the neck of the thigh-bone.' He observed that, 'women are much more likely to this species of fracture than men,' and that it 'seldom happens but at an advanced period of life.' He attributed the predilection for women to the 'comparative feebleness of the female constitution' and the relationship with old age to a deteriorating balance between 'absorption and deposition' (which he thought was due to diminishing arterial blood flow and unspecified 'absorbents').[1]

Cooper supplied the pathologic observation that bones become 'thin in their shell and spongy in their texture' and acquire 'a lightness and softness in the more advanced stages of life' such that 'the bones of old persons may be cut with a penknife. . .' He added,

> 'That this state of bone, in old age, favours much the production of fractures, is shown by the slightest causes often producing them. In London, the most frequent source of this accident is from a person, when walking on the edge of the elevated footpath, slipping upon the carriage pavement; and though it be a descent of only a few inches, yet from its occurring so suddenly and unexpectedly, it produces a fracture of the neck of the thigh-bone.'[1]

It was more than a century later when reports began to relate pathologic findings specifically to clinical conditions of fracture and postulated causal mechanisms. Albright et al[2] laid the groundwork for much subsequent work when they published findings on 40 cases of 'post-menopausal osteoporosis.' These authors characterized the dynamic process of bone formation and resorption and clarified the distinction between 'atrophy' of fully developed bone that produced a 'rarefied skeleton,' which they designated osteoporosis, and inadequate mineralization of bone matrix, osteomalacia. All the women in this series were under the age of 65 years and had experienced physiologic or 'artificial' menopause. Fractures were predominantly of the spine and were characterized by acute onset of localized back pain following minor trauma and were confirmed as vertebral deformities by radiologic examination. The report represented the first clear link between osteoporotic fracture and estrogen status.

Despite the insight that estrogen deficiency precipitated what appeared to be a pathologic deficit in bone, agreement was far from complete on the exact nature of the condition. Debate ensued whether osteoporosis, particularly among older women, actually constituted a disease. Newton-John and Morgan[3] chastised Albright for suggesting osteoporosis represented an abnormality. Following a review of 30 publications, they argued that all persons lost bone with age and that fracture-prone, 'thin bones' were an expected consequence of 'senescence,' not a disease due to excessive bone loss. They demonstrated that loss of bone mineral was universal among both older women and men and that fracture rates increased in concert with these losses of bone. They argued that 'thin bones' were a product, not of increased loss, but of 'less bone than average to start with.'[3] It turned out that both sets of observations had merit. The rapid loss of bone in women following menopause is crucial to development of osteoporosis as is the ongoing age-related loss; the latter is most likely to lead to compromised bone mass when peak, young adult levels are low.

Recent years have seen progress in clarifying the nature of osteoporosis, its pathophysiology, antecedent risks, and the relationship to fracture. However, some conceptual uncertainties remain. A watershed report issued by the World Health Organization (WHO) in 1994[4] has provided a useful framework for characterizing the problem and highlighted continuing challenges. The WHO study group acknowledged ongoing confusion, noting,

> 'the term osteoporosis is commonly used without a clear indication of its meaning. For example, it may describe both clinical end result (fracture) and the process that gives rise to fracture. As a disease process, it causes a decrease in bone density that is a major contributing factor to the increased risk of fracture.'

From the report came a definition that accommodated both perspectives. Osteoporosis is

> 'a disease characterised by low bone mass and micro-architectural deterioration of bone tissue, leading to enhanced bone fragility and a consequent increase in fracture risk.'

The group also recognized the challenge that lay in how best to characterize the vulnerable or high risk patient. One approach classifies the problem according to the mineral content of bone. The advantage in this lies in the availability of technology to accurately assess bone mineral density. Standards can be devised, populations measured and distributions of values described. Osteoporosis can then be defined by bone mineral values that occur at the low end of the population distribution. The primary limitation to this approach is the fact that bone mass, although primary, is not the only factor that contributes to bone fragility. The architecture of bone and rate of turnover are also part of the mix. These qualities are not readily assessed by the techniques at hand.

A second approach is to view the problem from the perspective of fracture risk. Although this idea has the merit of targeting the outcome of importance (fracture), it still requires some measurement on which to base such risk. The study group was forced to return to bone density as the best available assessment method. However, it was evident that there was no clear threshold or cut-point of bone mineral density that divides those who fracture from those who do not. Fractures occur over a range of bone densities and any cut-point is arbitrary. Misclassification is inevitable; some fractures will occur among those classified as low in risk and not all those in the high risk group will suffer fractures. Acknowledging all this, the study group selected a diagnostic guide that characterized osteoporosis based on a comparison of bone mineral density values against a standard of healthy young women. They estimated that:

'A measured value of bone mineral density more than 2.5 standard deviations below the mean for young healthy adult women at any site (spine, hip or mid radius) identifies 30% of all post-menopausal women having osteoporosis, more than half of whom will have sustained a prior fracture of the proximal femur, spine, distal forearm, proximal humerus or pelvis.'

Four categories were provided to guide diagnosis and further discussion. These are displayed in Table 1.1.

THE BONE DENSITY PERSPECTIVE

With the promulgation of the WHO guidelines, bone mineral density (BMD) has become the central arbiter of osteoporosis. The measure represents the average concentration of mineral (primarily calcium hydroxyapatite) per unit area of bone. The amount of mineral is, indeed, the most potent predictor of bone strength, although, as noted, other factors such as bone size and cross-sectional area (larger is stronger) as well as micro-architecture, also contribute to fractural resistance.

Decreased bone mineral content has long been recognized from plain radiographic examinations. However, while severe cases of osteoporosis are evident from these, such films are not sufficiently sensitive to identify less obvious, yet clinically important, cases of low bone density. Non-invasive, accurate quantitative techniques for determining bone mineral content have

Table 1.1	Diagnostic categories for osteoporosis based on WHO criteria
Category	**Definition by bone density**
Normal	A value for BMD that is not more than 1 SD below the young adult mean value
Osteopenia	A value for BMD that lies between 1 SD and 2.5 SD below the young adult mean value
Osteoporosis	A value for BMD that is more than 2.5 SD below the young adult mean value
Severe osteoporosis (established)	A value for BMD more than 2.5 SD below the young adult mean value in the presence of one or more fragility fractures

BMD = bone mineral density; SD = standard deviation.

become available, including single- and dual-energy X-ray absorptiometry (SXA, DXA) techniques as well as quantitative computed tomography (QCT). All three employ radiation to determine the mineral content of either a specific area (SXA and DXA) or volume of bone (QCT). The latest SXA and DXA scans are highly accurate, take only minutes to perform and subject patients to a very low radiation dose. (See Table 1.2.) They have the disadvantage of producing only two-dimensional estimates of density, however, so that bones of greater size/thickness may appear by artefact to have greater density. QCT, although providing a true measure of mineral content per unit volume, requires greater amounts of radiation exposure, is more time consuming, and generally more costly than X-ray absorptiometry. Quantitative ultrasound (QUS), a technology that utilizes variable sound wave transmission as a means of ascertaining bone density, is seeing increasing use as a lower cost, radiation-free method of measuring the mineral content at peripheral locations such as the heel and tibia.

The capacity to produce a spectrum of quantitative values for bone mass has been a major advance but still begs the question of how to determine when a result is low. A standard is required against which to compare values. Results of individual BMD determinations are thus presented not only as grams per square centimeter but in relation to one of two standards. The first is the mean value for a population of persons of the same age and sex, known as a Z-score, the second is the mean for a population of healthy young adults with optimal bone density, the T-score. The WHO definition of osteoporosis employs this latter measure. A BMD value that falls below 2.5 standard deviations (SD) from the young adult mean denotes osteoporosis, while a value between -1.0 SD and -2.5 SD is indicative of osteopenia.

Table 1.2   Summary of common techniques for assessment of bone mass

	Site	Scan time (min)	Precision error (%)	Approximate radiation exposure (mrem)
Peripheral DXA and SXA	Radius calcaneus	5–15	1–3	1
DXA	Spine, hip, whole body	5–10	1–2	1–5
Quantitative computed tomography (QCT)	Spine	10–30	2–4	50
Radiographic absorptiometry	Hands	5–10	1–2	5
Quantitative ultrasound (QUS)	Calcaneus, tibia	5–10	3–4	0

The skeletal sites most commonly assessed for bone density correspond with those that are most subject to fracture (i.e. the hip, spine and wrist), although, as noted, the heel (calcaneus) is also used for both DXA and QUS. Several practical problems of interpretation arise. Determinations obtained from anterior-posterior scans of the spine may include posterior vertebral elements and artefacts due to degenerative arthritis, and falsely elevated estimates of bone density can result. (Lateral views are preferred.) In addition, an individual's BMD can vary across measurement sites. A T-score may be in the 'osteoporotic' range when obtained at the spine but only 'osteopenic' when measured at the hip. Some consider values from the hip as most important, and the standard that defines osteoporosis. Others take any T-score site below −2.5 as a sufficient basis to make the diagnosis.[5] As multiple instruments have become available for BMD assessment, it is also apparent that there is considerable within-site variation in results. Estimates of density in the same spine or wrist can differ substantially not only with the technology (DXA vs QCT vs QUS) but with the same type of instruments produced by different manufacturers.[5]

THE FRACTURE PERSPECTIVE

There are, at first sight, several advantages in restricting the definition of osteoporosis to individuals who have sustained typical age-related fractures. These fractures comprise discrete clinical events, which can be diagnosed using relatively simple clinical and investigative algorithms. Such definitions would obviate the need to select a threshold value of bone density from a continuously rising gradient of risk, below which a disease process could be assigned. There are also disadvantages to this approach. First, the pathogenesis of fracture of the hip, spine and wrist entails a complex interplay between bone strength and trauma.[6] Although reduced bone density is a risk factor for fractures at each of these three sites, so are the pattern and severity of trauma. Second, while radiographic classification systems are widely available for hip and wrist fractures, the definition of prevalent and incident vertebral deformities remains highly contentious.[7] Finally, in a disorder for which preventive strategies are likely to yield greater dividends than therapeutic strategies in the general population, it seems prudent to include a classification category in which the risk factor (low bone density) might be present, but fracture might not yet have occurred.

Definition of fracture

The gold standard for fracture definition is radiological. Although the clinical features of osteoporotic fractures provide important indications as to the underlying diagnosis, fractures of the hip, distal forearm and spine require radiographic confirmation.

1. Hip fracture

The proximal portion of the femur includes the femoral head, neck and trochanteric region. The capsule of the hip joint extends from the acetabular margin to the intertrochanteric ridge. The principal blood supply to the femoral head and neck is provided by branches of the medial and lateral circumflex arteries, which form a vascular ring around the femoral neck. Hip fractures may be classified as intracapsular or extra-capsular. These are illustrated in Figure 1.1. Intracapsular fractures are usually classified according to the Garden scale: Type 1 incomplete, Type 2 complete without displacement, Type 3 complete with partial displacement and Type 4 complete with full displacement.[8,9] Extra-capsular fractures may be intertrochanteric or subtrochanteric. They are classified[10] according to stability (stable/unstable) and displacement (present/absent). These classification systems have a major influence on the choice of orthopedic interventions, such as internal fixation and arthroplasty. Whether the etiology of the two fractures also differs remains contentious. Some, but not all, studies have suggested that osteoporosis plays a greater role in causing extra-capsular fractures.[11]

2. Distal forearm fracture

The most common distal forearm fracture is Colles' fracture. This fracture lies within one inch of the wrist joint margin, is associated with dorsal angulation and displacement of the distal fragment of the radius and with a fracture of the ulnar styloid. The reverse injury, known as Smith's fracture, usually follows a forcible flexion injury to the wrist; it is relatively uncommon and tends to occur in young adults following major trauma.[12]

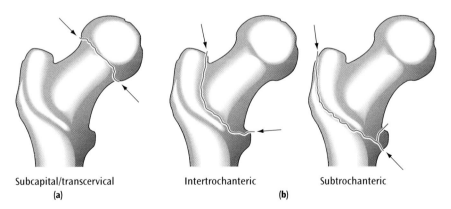

| Subcapital/transcervical | Intertrochanteric | Subtrochanteric |
| (a) | (b) | |

Figure 1.1

Classification of hip fracture: (a) subcapital/transcervical; (b) intertrochanteric, subtrochanteric.

3. Vertebral fracture

Vertebral fracture has been the most difficult osteoporosis-related fracture to define. The vertebral deformities that result from osteoporosis are usually classified into three forms: crush (involving compression of the entire vertebral body), wedge (in which there is anterior collapse), and end plate (where there is relative maintenance of anterior and posterior heights with central compression of the end plate regions). The difficulty in deciding whether a vertebra is deformed results from variation in shape of vertebral bodies both within the spine and between individuals. Initial studies of vertebral osteoporosis utilized subjective methods of defining the radiographic appearance of individual vertebral bodies. Such qualitative approaches[13] often led to within- and between-observer disagreements as to the presence or absence of deformity. This difficulty resulted in attempts to quantify deformity using measurements of vertebral dimensions. The earliest of these morphometric approaches measured vertebral height directly and defined abnormality according to some absolute reduction in height.[14] However, vertebral height is closely correlated with body height, making this approach inappropriate. A more complex alternative is measurement of the anterior, posterior and mid-vertebral heights, with deformity defined according to some threshold value. For example, a mild vertebral deformity might be defined as a 15% or greater reduction in the ratio of anterior to posterior height for a given vertebral body and a severe deformity as one with a 25% or greater reduction in the same ratio.[15] The problem here is that each vertebral body in the thoraco-lumbar spine has a unique shape and these site-specific differences are not taken into account.

More recently, morphometric approaches have entailed the same measurements but adopted different algorithms for the definition of abnormality.[16,17] Ratios have been calculated between anterior, posterior and mid-vertebral heights, corresponding to wedge, end plate and crush deformities. Each of these ratios, for each vertebral level, is normally distributed in the general population. The normal ranges are estimated from a radiographic population survey, and cut-off values for each type of deformity are arbitrarily assigned to points on the distribution of these ratios. Thus, mild (or grade 1) wedge deformity according to one of these algorithms is defined by a ratio of anterior to posterior height falling more than three standard deviations below the vertebra-specific population mean. Severe deformity (grade 2) is defined by a ratio falling more than four standard deviations below this value.[18]

In an effort to clarify confusion that may come from the multiple approaches, the International Osteoporosis Foundation and European Society of Musculoskeletal Radiology has begun a vertebral fracture initiative which aims to standardize the radiographic assessment of vertebral fracture; establish comparisons between semi-quantitative and quantitative techniques; review the position of lateral spine DXA imaging; and present criteria for the adequate reporting of radiographic vertebral deformities.[19]

Fracture burden

The impact of osteoporosis in terms of fracture occurrence is best assessed by calculating the lifetime risk of hip, spine and wrist fractures among men and women in the general population.[20] The lifetime risk of hip fracture in North American men and women aged 50 years is 17.5% and 6%, respectively. This contrasts with risks of 15.6% and 5.6% for clinically diagnosed vertebral fractures and 16% and 2.5% for distal forearm fractures, in white women and men, respectively. The lifetime risk of any of the three fractures is 39.7% for women and 13.1% for men from the age of 50 years onwards. On this basis, around 60,000 hip fractures, 40,000 clinically diagnosed vertebral fractures and 50,000 distal forearm fractures occur in British women each year.

Ultimately, the probability of fracture in any bone will depend upon the force applied to the bone and its strength.[21] All bones will fracture if sufficient trauma is applied to them, though the level of trauma required to fracture pathologically weak bone may be low. The variable shape, composition and load-bearing properties of bones in the skeleton require that etiological models for fracture are site-specific. Thus, for example, external trauma through a fall may play a greater role in causing distal forearm fractures than vertebral fractures.

Although pathological processes may sometimes weaken a bone to such an extent that it fractures following forces from gravity and muscle contraction, the majority of age-related fractures are associated with an injury. This most frequently takes the form of a fall from standing height or less. However, only 5–6 in every 100 falls of this type in elderly people culminate in a fracture, and the potential energy generated by such falls far exceeds the breaking strength of most bones in the body.[22] These observations highlight the importance of a variety of energy-absorbing mechanisms that operate to prevent bony injury. These mechanisms include the padding effect of adipose and other soft

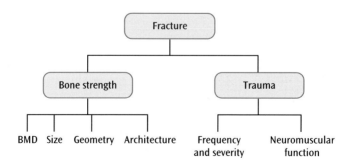

Figure 1.2

Determinants of fracture risk.

tissues, as well as neuromuscular reflexes, which absorb the forces generated during a fall.

Clearly, qualitative aspects of bone structure, such as geometry, architecture and size, influence bone strength. Properties such as internal trabecular connectivity, repair of bone tissue microdamage, and impairment of mineralization all contribute to the mechanical strength of bone and thereby to the potential for fracture in the event of a specified level of trauma.[23] However, bone mineral density accounts for 75–90% of the variance in bone strength. Moreover, of all of these factors, it is only bone mass quantified as bone mineral density, which can currently be measured with precision and accuracy. Consequently, it is this measurement that forms the basis for the diagnosis of osteoporosis.

REFERENCES

1. Cooper AP. *A Treatise on Dislocations and Fractures of the Joints*, 2nd edn. London: Longman, Hurst, Rees, Orme and Browne, 1823.

2. Albright F, Smith P, Richardson A. Postmenopausal osteoporosis; its clinical features. *JAMA* 1941;**116**: 2465–74.

3. Newton-John HF, Morgan DB. Osteoporosis: disease or senescence? *Lancet* 1968;**1**:232–3.

4. World Health Organization. *Assessment of fracture risk and its application to screening for osteoporosis. Technical Report Series 843.* Geneva: WHO, 1994.

5. Cummings SR, Bates D, Black DM. Clinical use of bone densitometry: scientific review. *JAMA* 2002;**288**: 1889–97.

6. Nevitt MC, Cummings BR et al. Type of fall and risk of hip and wrist fractures: the study of osteoporotic fractures. *J Am Geriatr Soc* 1993;**41**: 1226–34.

7. National Osteoporosis Foundation Working Group. Assessing vertebral fractures. *J Bone Miner Res* 1995;**10**: 518–23.

8. Garden RS. Low angle fixation in fractures of the femoral neck. *J Bone Joint Surg* 1961;**43B**:647–63.

9. Garden RS. The structure and function of the proximal end of the femur. *J Bone Joint Surg* 1961;**43B**: 576–89.

10. Evans EM. Trochanteric fractures. *J Bone Joint Surg* 1951;**33B**:192–204.

11. Melton LJ. Epidemiology of fractures. In: Riggs BL, Melton LJ, eds. *Osteoporosis: Etiology, Diagnosis and Management.* New York: Raven Press, 1988:133–54.

12. Benjamin A. Injuries of the forearm. In: Wilson JW, ed. *Watson–Jones Fractures and Joint Injuries*, Vol. 2. Edinburgh: Churchill Livingstone, 1982: 650–709.

13. Iskrant AP, Smith RW. Osteoporosis in women 45 years and over related to subsequent fractures. *Public Health Rep* 1969;**84**:33–8.

14. Gallagher JC, Hedlund LR, Stoner S, Merger C. Vertebral morphometry: Normative data. *Bone Miner* 1988;**4**: 189–96.

15. Melton LJ, Kan SH, Frye MA et al. Epidemiology of vertebral fractures in women. *Am J Epidemiol* 1989;**129**: 1000–11.

16. Eastell R, Cedel SL, Wahner HW et al. Classification of vertebral fractures. *J Bone Miner Res* 1991;**6**: 207–15.

17. Black DM, Cummings SR, Stone K et al. A new approach to defining normal vertebral dimensions. *J Bone Miner Res* 1991;**6**:883–92.

18. Melton LJ, Lane AW, Cooper C et al. Prevalence and incidence of vertebral deformities. *Osteoporos Int* 1993;**3**: 113–19.

19. International Osteoporosis Foundation. In: Genant HK, Jergas M, Van Kuijk C, eds. *Vertebral Fracture Initiative Resource Document.* Geneva: IOF, 2003:1–36.
20. Melton LJ, Chrischilles EA, Cooper C et al. How many women have osteoporosis? *J Bone Miner Res* 1993;7: 1005–10.
21. Cooper C, Melton LJ. Magnitude and impact of osteoporosis and fractures. In: Marcus R, Feldman D, Kelsey J, eds. *Osteoporosis.* San Diego: Academic Press, 1996:419–34.
22. Gillespie LD, Gillespie WJ, Robertson MC, Lamb SE, Cumming RG, Rowe BH. Interventions for preventing falls in elderly people (Cochrane Review). In: *The Cochrane Library, Issue 1.* Chichester, UK: Wiley, 2004.
23. Heaney RP. Qualitative factors in osteoporotic fracture: the state of the question. In: Christiansen C, ed. *Osteoporosis 1987, I. Proceedings of the International Symposium on Osteoporosis, Denmark.* Copenhagen: Osteoporosis ApS, 1987:281–7.

2
Epidemiology

L Joseph Melton, III

INTRODUCTION

Why should clinicians be concerned about osteoporosis and its related fractures? First, osteoporosis is a major public health problem and one that affects
a large segment of the population. Although now mainly a concern in Western
Europe and North America, osteoporosis is a global medical problem that will
increase in significance with the growing elderly population worldwide.
Because the disorder is so common, physicians of almost every specialty will
see patients with osteoporosis in their practices, though most of them may go
unrecognized and untreated. Many of these patients will experience fractures
as a result of their osteoporosis. Not only will the attending physicians have to
manage this acute event, but they will need to deal with the adverse outcomes
that can ensue, including death, disability and a reduced quality of life. Finally,
the care of osteoporotic fractures is very expensive, and costs will continue to
rise as fractures increase in the future. All of these aspects of the osteoporosis
problem are reviewed in the sections below. This epidemiologic information
provides some context for the detailed assessment of key issues in the diagnosis
and management of osteoporosis that are covered in subsequent chapters.

FREQUENCY OF OSTEOPOROSIS

Although osteoporosis is a systemic disease, patterns of bone loss differ by
skeletal site. In the appendicular skeleton, bone loss begins around the time of
menopause in women and at a comparable age in men.[1] At the femoral neck,
on the other hand, bone loss begins before age 20 years and is approximately
linear over life in men and women of all races (Figure 2.1). Given these
patterns, changes in the prevalence of osteoporosis with age are predictable.
Thus, among white women in Rochester, Minnesota, the prevalence of osteoporosis at the femoral neck increases from 10% at 50–59 years of age to 66%
at age 80 years and over, and from 6% to 78% at the total wrist site, but only
from 2% to 4% across this age-range at the anterior-posterior (AP) lumbar

spine.[1] (The appearance of little decline in BMD of the lumbar spine with aging is largely an artefact of age-related increases in aortic calcification and vertebral osteophytosis on dual-energy X-ray absorptiometry (DXA) scans of the AP spine. Lateral spine scans show substantial age-related bone loss in older women and men.)

Data from the third National Health and Nutrition Examination Survey (NHANES), a probability sample of the entire US population, reveal that the overall prevalence of osteoporosis at the femoral neck is 17% among postmenopausal white women.[2] This compares with a 21% figure among postmenopausal women in Sweden[3] but only 8% among white women in Canada.[4] Such differences could help account for the fact that hip fracture incidence is greater in Sweden and lower in Canada than in the USA.[5] The age-adjusted prevalence of osteoporosis among postmenopausal white women in Rochester is 33% at the total wrist and 8% at the AP lumbar spine. In the Canadian Multicentre Osteoporosis Study, the prevalence of osteoporosis at the lumbar spine was estimated at 12%.[4] If, however, DXA scans are made of the lateral spine instead, the prevalence of lumbar osteoporosis among Rochester women is 33%. Based on conventional scans of the total hip, total wrist and AP spine, an estimated 35% of postmenopausal white women have osteoporosis of at least one site according to the WHO definition.[1]

Osteoporosis and race/ethnicity

It is unclear exactly how osteoporosis should be defined in nonwhite women. Based on the normal values for white women from NHANES, the prevalence of

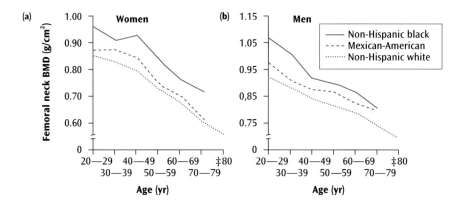

Figure 2.1

Mean bone mineral density (BMD) of the femoral neck by age for US men and women of different ethnic groups. (Reproduced with permission from Looker et al, 1995.[6])

osteoporosis at the femoral neck among postmenopausal African-American women in the USA is just 6%, while the prevalence among Hispanic women is 14%.[2] These results are consistent with the observation that hip fracture rates are lower in African-Americans and in most populations of Spanish heritage compared to persons of Northern European origin.[5] Data from the Japanese Population-Based Osteoporosis Study indicate that the prevalence of osteo-porosis at the femoral neck is only 12% in Asian women, whereas the preva-lence of osteoporosis in the lumbar spine is as high as or higher than that seen in white women.[7] Consistent with these findings, vertebral fractures are almost as frequent among Asian women as they are in white women, whereas hip fractures are much less common.[5] However, the latter difference has also been attributed to a lower risk of falling among Asian women. It is important to recognize that patterns of bone loss, and therefore osteoporosis prevalence, may vary between different populations of Asian or African heritage so these groups cannot necessarily be considered homogeneous from the point of view of osteoporosis diagnosis and management.

Osteoporosis and sex

Although volumetric bone density (g/cm^3) is similar in women and men, two-dimensional DXA scans do not fully correct for the larger size of men's bones so their areal BMD (g/cm^2) values appear to be greater. As a consequence, the prevalence of osteoporosis in men by DXA is less than in women, despite the fact that aging men of all races lose bone at rates approaching those for compa-rable women.[6] Based on the same absolute bone density cut-off level for men as for white women (0.56 g/cm^2 for femoral neck BMD), the prevalence of osteoporosis at the femoral neck among white, Hispanic and African-American men aged 50 years and over in the USA is only 4%, 2% and 3%, respectively.[2] Similarly, data from Great Britain suggest that about 6% of men have hip BMD more than 2.5 standard deviations (SD) below the normal mean for young women compared to 22% of older British women.[8]

However, osteoporosis prevalence estimates increase somewhat when male normal values are used. Thus, when NHANES rates were recalculated on the basis of femoral neck BMD levels more than 2.5 SD below the mean for young white men (0.59 g/cm^2), the higher mean value caused the prevalence esti-mates for white, Hispanic and African-American men $\geq$ 50 years of age to increase to 7%, 3% and 5%, respectively.[2] The comparable figure for men in the Canadian Multicentre Osteoporosis Study was almost 5%.[4] In that investi-gation, the prevalence of osteoporosis at the femoral neck increased from about 3% in men aged 50–59 years to around 14% at age 80 years and over. The prevalence of osteoporosis at the AP lumbar spine is 1% among white men 50 years of age or over in Rochester,[1] 3% among men in Canada[4] and 6% among French men.[9]

FREQUENCY OF FRACTURES

The fracture sites most closely associated with osteoporosis are those of the hip, spine and distal forearm, although almost all fractures among elderly women and men are partly related to low bone mass. The etiology of these fractures is discussed in Chapter 3.

Hip fracture

The complex pathophysiology of hip fractures results in an exponential increase in incidence with age, from 2 per 100,000 per year among white women less than 35 years of age to 3 per 100 per year among women 85 years old or over in the USA (Figure 2.2). Among older individuals, the incidence of hip fractures in men is about half that in women. This is because men are less likely to fall, the precipitating event for most of these fractures, and they are less likely to attain the very low BMD levels associated with the greatest fracture risk in women. In addition, there are fewer elderly men so about 80% of all hip fractures occur among women. Hip fracture rates are typically much less in nonwhite populations.[5] The explanation for this observation remains obscure but may relate to a lower risk of falling since bone density measurements are similar in white and nonwhite women and men after correction for differences in bone size. Even less obvious is the reason for substantial geographic differences in hip fracture incidence among white populations,[5] although hip bone density is lowest in the Southern region of the USA,[10] where hip fracture risk is highest,[11] and higher in Southern Europe,[12] where hip fracture risk is lowest.[13]

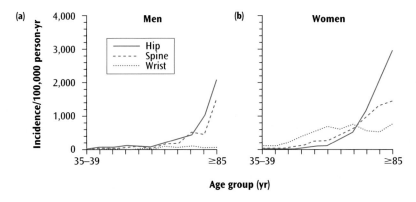

Figure 2.2

Age-specific incidence rates for hip, vertebral (spine), and distal forearm (wrist) fractures in Rochester, Minnesota, men and women. (Reproduced with permission from Cooper and Melton, 1992[14].)

Vertebral fracture

There is also substantial geographic variation in vertebral fractures and this may also be explained in part by differences in the prevalence of osteoporosis.[14] However, methodologic problems are paramount in this instance because there is no universally accepted definition of vertebral fracture and because a substantial proportion of these fractures are asymptomatic. Thus, the number of people affected depends largely on the criterion used for diagnosis. By one approach, an estimated 20–25% of postmenopausal white women have at least one moderate vertebral deformity on spine radiographs, while the prevalence of more severe vertebral deformities is about 10%.[15] The latter are more likely to produce chronic symptoms and account for the majority of vertebral fractures that come to clinical attention. Thus, the annual incidence of clinically diagnosed vertebral fractures among postmenopausal white women in the USA (5 per 1000) is only a third of the total estimated incidence (18 per 1000) as judged by vertebral morphometry.[16] In prospective studies in Europe, the annual incidence of morphometrically detected vertebral fractures is about 11 per 1000.[17,18]

Despite these problems, it is clear that the incidence of vertebral fracture increases with age (Figure 2.2). The age-related increase in falls plays a role, but most of these fractures can be linked to excessive compressive loads on the vertebrae that result from everyday activities. At younger ages, vertebral fractures are almost as common in men as in women,[19,20] but some of those in men may be attributable to occupational injuries or trauma. Likewise, the prevalence of vertebral fractures among Asians may be nearly as high as in whites, despite their lower hip fracture rates, but vertebral fractures appear to be less common among black and Hispanic men and women.[5] Again, the explanation for these differences is unclear at present.

Wrist fracture

Distal forearm fractures almost always result from a fall but, unlike hip fractures, these falls are typically forward on the outstretched arm. Consequently, forearm fractures are more common among younger and healthier individuals, and a greater proportion of them occur out of doors.[15] In most early studies, incidence rates in women increased linearly to around age 65 years and then stabilized, which was attributed to the fact that elderly women with slow gait and impaired neuromuscular co-ordination are more likely to fall backward on their hip rather than forward on their wrist. However, more recent studies show that incidence rates are now continuing to rise among elderly women.[21–23] In men, the incidence of forearm fractures is low and increases very little with aging (Figure 2.2), so that the majority of such fractures occur in women. Like most other osteoporotic fractures, forearm fracture incidence is lower in nonwhite compared to white populations, and the variation in rates from one geographic area to another is generally in parallel with hip fracture incidence.[5] Forearm fractures are important because they may be a harbinger of subsequent hip fracture risk.

Lifetime fracture risk

One measure of interest to patients and clinicians alike is the probability of experiencing a fracture over an average lifetime. Because women live longer than men, the lifetime risk of hip fracture from age 50 years onward has been estimated at 17% for white women but only 6% for white men in the USA.[16] However, lifetime risk in both sexes will increase as life expectancy continues to improve. Thus, in a similar analysis, the lifetime risk of a hip fracture was 14% and 5%, respectively, in Swedish women and men, but this rose to 23% and 11%, respectively, when projected improvements in mortality were accounted for.[24] If, in addition, age-adjusted hip fracture incidence rates were to rise by just 1% annually in Sweden, the lifetime risk could increase to an incredible 35% in women and 17% in men.

This compares with current lifetime risk estimates of 16% and 5% for clinically diagnosed vertebral fractures and 16% and 2% for distal forearm fractures in white women and men, respectively; the lifetime risk of any one of these three fractures is 40% for women and 13% for men from age 50 years onward in the USA.[16] In Australia, the lifetime risk of any fracture is 44% for women and 27% for men.[25] In Great Britain, the lifetime risk of a hip fracture among 50-year-old men is 3%, compared to 14% for British women of comparable age; because lifetime risk depends on life expectancy as well as fracture incidence, however, the lifetime risk of hip fracture in British women could rise to 24% by 2050 if life expectancy continues to increase.[26] It is obvious from these figures that osteoporotic fractures pose a threat to a substantial portion of the adult population.

FRACTURE-RELATED MORBIDITY

Functional impairment is widespread among the elderly but, even allowing for this, an estimated 7% of women with fractures of the hip, spine or distal forearm become dependent in the basic activities of daily living.[27] Hip fractures contribute the most to this burden (Figure 2.3). Hip fracture patients are at high risk of acute complications such as pressure sores, pneumonia and urinary tract infections, but the most important adverse outcome is impairment in the ability to walk. By one year following a hip fracture, only 40–79% of patients have regained their prior ambulatory function, and less than half of them have returned to their prefracture status with respect to the activities of daily living.[28]

Indeed, hip fracture patients are as likely to experience impaired ambulation, other functional deficits and depression as are the victims of a stroke.[29] Rehabilitation efforts often have limited success in these patients. Consequently, an estimated 10% of women may become functionally dependent following hip fracture, and 19% require long-term nursing home care.[27] Nearly 140,000 nursing home admissions each year are attributable to hip fractures in the USA alone,[30] but even those individuals who remain independent may experience a substantial reduction in their quality of life.

New compression fractures may produce severe back pain that lasts for weeks or months, but the long-term impact of vertebral fractures is more difficult to quantify. Only about a third of affected women have the severe (or multiple) vertebral deformities most likely to produce chronic symptoms, including height loss, kyphosis, postural changes and persistent pain that interferes with daily activities.[32] While these fractures are rarely the direct cause of institutionalization,[27] their adverse influence on most activities of daily living is almost as great as that seen for hip fractures (Table 2.1). Moreover, not only physical function but self-esteem, body image and mood are also negatively affected by vertebral fractures.[33] This is largely responsible for the reduced quality of life observed among women with osteoporosis generally.

By contrast, few forearm fracture patients are disabled,[27] but nearly half report unsatisfactory function at six months. A third or more have hand pain or weakness and there is a substantial risk of algodystrophy, as well as an increased likelihood of post-traumatic arthritis.[28] Indeed, forearm fractures account for 39% of all physical therapy sessions attributable to osteoporotic fractures in the USA.[30] In addition, forearm fractures are as disabling as hip

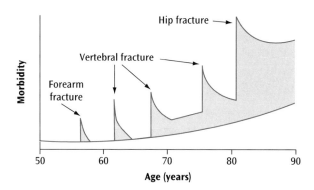

Figure 2.3

Schematic representation of the morbidity associated with different osteoporotic fractures with age. Distal forearm (Colles') fractures commonly occur in women in their mid 50s and have short-term sequelae; repeated vertebral fractures occurring at a later age may give rise to permanent morbidity; hip fractures occur at age 80 years on average and usually result in permanent morbidity. (Reproduced with permission from Kanis and Johnell, 1999.[31])

Table 2.1 Physical and functional impairment associated with selected minimal trauma fractures among women in Rancho Bernardo, CA

	Odds of impairment[*]		
	Hip fracture	Spine fracture	Wrist fracture
Movements			
Bend	2.7	3.1	1.2
Lift	1.1	3.4	1.3
Reach	1.5	0.7	1.8
Walk	3.6	2.7	1.6
Climb stairs	2.6	2.2	1.8
Descend stairs	4.1	4.2	2.5
Get into/out of car	1.3	2.1	1.3
Activities			
Put socks on	1.6	1.7	1.1
Cook meals	11.1	6.9	10.2
Shop	4.6	5.2	3.3
Heavy housework	2.8	2.1	1.6

Source: Modified with permission from Greendale et al.[34]
[*]Likelihood of having the impaired activity following fracture after adjusting for age, body mass index, estrogen use, visual impairment and reduced mental status.

fractures with respect to some specific activities of daily living, such as preparing meals.[34] It is worth noting that the burden of managing these impairments can fall on the attending physician as well as the patient. Although the overall impact on patient quality of life is far less than a hip fracture, distal forearm and other limb fractures contribute disproportionately to osteoporosis-related morbidity in middle-aged women and men.[35]

FRACTURE-RELATED MORTALITY

The influence of osteoporotic fractures on survival varies with the type of fracture. Hip fractures are the most serious, leading to an overall reduction of 12–20% from expected survival.[15] Relative mortality is increased from 1.2-fold to 2.4-fold,[36,37] but differences in these figures are partly a function of the duration of follow-up. The hazard of death is increased over 10-fold in the first weeks following a hip fracture and then diminishes over time (Figure 2.4), although the death rate may remain elevated for a number of years. Survival decreases with age and is worse among men than women. Moreover, the proportion of remaining years of life lost is greater in men with a hip fracture.[38] This sex difference appears to arise from the greater frequency of chronic

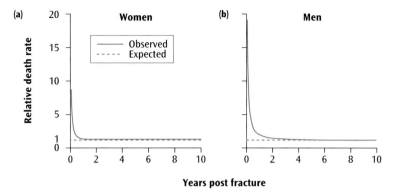

Figure 2.4

Relative death rate among Rochester, Minnesota, women (a) and men (b) by time following hip fracture compared with that expected for West North Central US residents. (Modified with permission from Springer-Verlag, from Melton et al, 1998.[43])

disease among men who sustain a hip fracture.[39] Thus, while some deaths are attributable to acute complications, the majority appear to be due to serious coexisting illnesses.[37]

Patients who sustain a distal forearm fracture experience no excess mortality,[16] but other limb fractures have been linked to an increased risk of death.[37,40] The death rate following vertebral fracture is 1.2 to 1.9 times greater than expected,[41] but most of these deaths occur some time after the initial fracture. Strong associations with specific causes of death have not been identified in patients with vertebral fractures, suggesting an indirect association with underlying comorbid conditions that may lead not only to death but also to osteoporosis. This is consistent with the observation that low bone density per se may be associated with excess mortality.[41] Nonetheless, deaths in one clinical trial were still increased in women with vertebral fractures compared to those with low bone mass even though patients with secondary osteoporosis had been excluded from the study.[42]

FRACTURE-RELATED COST

The cost of managing the large number of fractures that occur each year is great, as the average incremental direct medical expenditure in the year following fracture may exceed US $2000, with a median incremental cost for hip fractures alone of more than US $11,000.[44] These expenses are typically borne by society since nearly three-quarters of hip, spine and distal forearm fractures occur among patients 65 years old or over. Annual treatment costs for osteoporotic fractures in Australia totaled A $779 million,[45] while worldwide costs for hip fractures alone were estimated at US $34.9 billion in 1990.[31] Lost wages or reduced years of life are not the primary determinants of cost in these mostly elderly patients. Rather, expenses are mainly for inpatient medical services and nursing home care.

Direct expenditures for osteoporotic fractures in the USA in 1995 totaled US $13.8 billion, or US $17.5 billion in 2002.[30] This exceeds annual expenditures for breast and gynecologic malignancies combined but not those for cardiovascular disease.[46] Although hip fractures account for 63% of the total cost, the other fractures associated with osteoporosis are responsible for the majority of all fracture-related services except for nursing home and home health care.[30] It is also important to note that nonwhite women and men accounted for US $1 billion of the USA total, reinforcing the point that osteoporosis in other races cannot be ignored.

These costs can only increase in the future as the population ages. In the USA, for example, the number of persons aged 65 years and over is expected to rise from 32 million to 69 million between 1990 and 2050, while the number aged 85 years and over will increase from 3 million to 15 million. These demographic changes will cause a substantial increase in the number of affected women. Considering osteoporosis of the hip alone, an estimated 7.8 million women and 2.3 million men in the USA are affected today, but these figures could rise to 10.5 million and 3.3 million, respectively, by the year 2020.[47] Likewise, the demographic changes could lead to a doubling or tripling in the number of hip fractures in the USA by the year 2040,[5] with similar increases in Europe,[31] while a four-fold increase is expected in Australia.[48] (See Table 2.2.)

Table 2.2   Projected number of hip fractures worldwide in 2050 given different assumptions about changing incidence rates

	Number of fractures	
Scenario	Men	Women
1990 base case	338,000	917,000
2050 no change in incidence	1,381,000	3,112,000
2050 1% increase in incidence worldwide	2,509,000	5,653,000
2050 no change in North America/Europe but 2% increase elsewhere	3,905,000	8,430,000
2050 no change in North America/Europe but 3% increase elsewhere	6,794,000	14,516,000
2050 no change in North America/Europe but 4% increase elsewhere	11,916,000	25,305,000

Source: Modified with permission from Gullberg et al.[49]

Worldwide, the 323 million individuals aged 65 years and over in 1990 will grow to an estimated 1555 million by 2050, and this by itself could cause the number of hip fractures worldwide to increase from the estimated 1.7 million in 1990 to a projected 6.3 million in 2050.[15] If, in addition, hip fracture incidence rates increase by 1% annually, the projected number of fractures in 2050 could be 8.2 million (Table 2.2). If instead, incidence rates continue to stabilize in Europe and North America but increase by 3% annually in the other regions, the total number of hip fractures in the world each year could exceed 21 million by 2050.[49] In fact, increases of this magnitude in hip fracture incidence have been seen recently in some areas of the world.

CONCLUSIONS

Fractures, the clinical manifestation of osteoporosis, not only are extremely common but are also devastating both to the affected patients and to the societies that must bear the enormous cost of fracture treatment and subsequent disability. It has been estimated that in a 10-year period, postmenopausal white women in the USA will experience 5.2 million fractures of the hip, spine or distal forearm, which will lead to 2 million person-years of fracture-related disability and to over US $45 billion in direct medical expenditures.[50] These costs can only rise in the future as the population ages. If the impact of these fractures is to be reduced, increased attention must be given to the design and implementation of effective control programs. The issue is how to accomplish this at a socially acceptable cost. At present, only a minority of patients is treated for osteoporosis. It is important that prophylaxis in the future be directed at all of the fracture outcomes of osteoporosis.[35]

ACKNOWLEDGMENTS

This work was supported in part by research grants AG 04875, AR 27065 and AR 30582 from the National Institutes of Health, US Public Health Service.

The author would like to thank Mrs Mary Roberts for assistance in preparing the manuscript.

REFERENCES

1. Melton LJ III, Atkinson EJ, O'Connor MK et al. Bone density and fracture risk in men. *J Bone Miner Res* 1998; **13**:1915–23.

2. Looker AC, Orwoll ES, Johnston CC Jr et al. Prevalence of low femoral bone density in older US adults from NHANES III. *J Bone Miner Res* 1997; **12**:1761–8.

3. Kanis JA, Johnell O, Oden A et al. Risk of hip fracture according to the World Health Organization criteria for osteopenia and osteoporosis. *Bone* 2000;**27**:585–90.

4. Tenenhouse A, Joseph L, Kreiger N et al. Estimation of the prevalence of low bone density in Canadian women and men using a population-specific DXA reference standard: The Canadian Multicentre Osteoporosis Study (CaMos). *Osteoporos Int* 2000;**11**:897–4.

5. Melton LJ III. Epidemiology of fractures. In: Orwoll E, ed. *Osteoporosis in Men: The Effects of Gender on Skeletal Health*. San Diego: Academic Press, 1999:1–13.

6. Looker AC, Wahner HW, Dunn WL et al. Proximal femur bone mineral levels of US adults. *Osteoporos Int* 1995;**5**:389–409.

7. Iki M, Kagamimori S, Kagawa Y et al. Bone mineral density of the spine, hip and distal forearm in representative samples of the Japanese female population: Japanese Population-Based Osteoporosis (JPOS) Study. *Osteoporos Int* 2001;**12**:529–37.

8. Kanis JA, Melton LJ III, Christiansen C et al. The diagnosis of osteoporosis. *J Bone Miner Res* 1994;**9**:1137–41.

9. Szulc P, Marchand F, Duboeuf F, Delmas PD. Cross-sectional assessment of age-related bone loss in men: The MINOS Study. *Bone* 2000;**26**:123–9.

10. Looker AC, Wahner HW, Dunn WL et al. Updated data on proximal femur bone mineral levels of US adults. *Osteoporos Int* 1998;**8**:468–89.

11. Karagas MR, Baron JA, Barrett JA, Jacobsen SJ. Patterns of fracture among the United States elderly: Geographic and fluoride effects. *Ann Epidemiol* 1996;**6**:209–16.

12. Lunt M, Felsenberg D, Adams J et al. Population-based geographic variations in DXA bone density in Europe: The EVOS Study. *Osteoporos Int* 1997;**7**:175–89.

13. Elffors I, Allander E, Kanis JA et al. The variable incidence of hip fracture in southern Europe. The MEDOS Study. *Osteoporos Int* 1994; **4**:253–63.

14. Cooper C, Melton LJ III. Epidemiology of osteoporosis. *Trends Endocrinol Metabol* 1992;**3**:224–9.

15. Melton LJ III, Cooper C. Magnitude and impact of osteoporosis and fractures. In: Marcus R, Feldman D, Kelsey J, eds. *Osteoporosis*, Vol 1, 2nd edn. San Diego: Academic Press, 2001:557–67.

16. Cummings SR, Melton LJ III. Epidemiology and outcomes of osteoporotic fractures. *Lancet* 2002;**359**:1761–7.

17. Anonymous. Incidence of vertebral fracture in Europe: Results from the European Prospective Osteoporosis Study (EPOS). *J Bone Miner Res* 2002;**17**:716–24.

18. Van der Klift M, de Laet CEDH, McCloskey EV et al. The incidence of vertebral fractures in men and women: The Rotterdam Study. *J Bone Miner Res* 2002;**17**:1051–6.

19. O'Neill TW, Felsenberg D, Varlow J et al. The prevalence of vertebral deformity in European men and women: The European Vertebral Osteoporosis Study. *J Bone Miner Res* 1996;**11**:1010–18.

20. Davies KM, Stegman MR, Heaney RP, Recker RR. Prevalence and severity of vertebral fracture: The Saunders County Bone Quality Study. *Osteoporos Int* 1996;**6**:160–5.

21. Melton LJ III, Amadio PC Crowson CS, O'Fallon WM. Long-term trends

in the incidence of distal forearm fractures. *Osteoporos Int* 1998;**8:** 341–8.

22. Sanders KM, Seeman E, Ugoni AM et al. Age- and gender-specific rate of fractures in Australia: A population-based study. *Osteoporos Int* 1999; **10:**240–7.

23. O'Neill TW, Cooper C, Finn JD et al. Incidence of distal forearm fracture in British men and women. *Osteoporos Int* 2001;**12:**555–8.

24. Oden A, Dawson A, Dere W et al. Lifetime risk of hip fractures is under-estimated. *Osteoporos Int* 1998;**8:** 599–603.

25. Cooley H, Jones G. A population-based study of fracture incidence in Southern Tasmania: Lifetime fracture risk and evidence for geographic variations within the same country. *Osteoporos Int* 2001;**12:**124–30.

26. Cooper C. Epidemiology of osteoporosis. *Osteoporos Int* 1999;**9**(Suppl 2): S2–S8.

27. Chrischilles EA, Butler CD, Davis CS, Wallace RB. A model of lifetime osteoporosis impact. *Arch Intern Med* 1991; **151:**2026–32.

28. Greendale GA, Barrett-Connor E. Outcomes of osteoporotic fractures. In: Marcus R, Feldman D, Kelsey J, eds. *Osteoporosis*, Vol 1, 2nd edn. San Diego: Academic Press, 2001: 819–29.

29. Lieberman D, Friger M, Fried V et al. Characterization of elderly patients in rehabilitation: Stroke versus hip fracture. *Disabil Rehabil* 1999;**21:** 542–7.

30. Ray NF, Chan JK, Thamer M, Melton LJ III. Medical expenditures for the treatment of osteoporotic fractures in the United States in 1995: Report from the National Osteoporosis Foundation. *J Bone Miner Res* 1997; **12:**24–35.

31. Kanis JA, Johnell O. The burden of osteoporosis. *J Endocrinol Invest* 1999; **22:**583–8.

32. Ross PD. Clinical consequences of vertebral fractures. *Am J Med* 1997; **103(2A):**S30–S43.

33. Gold DT, Lyles KW, Shipp KM, Drezner MK. Osteoporosis and its nonskeletal consequences: Their impact on treatment decisions. In: Marcus R, Feldman D, Kelsey J, eds. *Osteoporosis*, Vol 2, 2nd edn. San Diego: Academic Press, 2001: 479–84

34. Greendale GA, Barrett-Connor E, Ingles S, Haile R. Late physical and functional effects of osteoporotic fracture in women: The Rancho Bernardo Study. *J Am Geriatr Soc* 1995;**43:**955–61.

35. Kanis JA, Oden A, Johnell O et al. The burden of osteoporotic fractures: A method for setting intervention thresholds. *Osteoporos Int* 2001;**12:** 417–27.

36. Cooper C, Atkinson EJ, Jacobsen SJ et al. Population-based study of survival after osteoporotic fractures. *Am J Epidemiol* 1993;**137:**1001–5.

37. Browner WS, Pressman AR, Nevitt MC, Cummings SR. Mortality following fractures in older women. The Study of Osteoporotic Fractures. *Arch Intern Med* 1996;**156:**1521–5.

38. Trombetti A, Herrmann F, Hoffmeyer P et al. Survival and potential years of life lost after hip fracture in men and age-matched women. *Osteoporos Int* 2002;**13:**731–7.

39. Poór G, Atkinson EJ, O'Fallon WM, Melton LJ III. Determinants of reduced survival following hip fractures in men. *Clin Orthop* 1995; **319:**260–5.

40. Center JR, Nguyen TV, Schneider D et al. Mortality after all major types of osteoporotic fracture in men and women: An observational study. *Lancet* 1999;**353:**878–82.

41. Melton LJ III. Excess mortality following vertebral fracture. *J Am Geriatr Soc* 2000;**48:**338–9.

42. Ensrud KE, Thompson DE, Cauley JA et al. Prevalent vertebral deformities predict mortality and hospitalization in older women with low bone mass. Fracture Intervention Trial Research Group. *J Am Geriatr Soc* 2000;**48:** 241–9.

43. Melton LJ III, Therneau TM, Larson DR. Long-term trends in hip fracture prevalence: The influence of hip fracture incidence and survival. *Osteoporos Int* 1998;**8**:68–74.

44. Gabriel SE, Tosteson ANA, Leibson CL et al. Direct medical costs attributable to osteoporotic fractures. *Osteoporos Int* 2002;**13**:323–30.

45. Randell A, Sambrook PN, Nguyen RV et al. Direct clinical and welfare costs of osteoporotic fractures in elderly men and women. *Osteoporos Int* 1995; **5**:427–32.

46. Hoerger TJ, Downs KE, Lakshmanan MC et al. Healthcare use among US women aged 45 and older: Total costs and costs for selected postmenopausal health risks. *J Womens Health Gender-Based Med* 1999;**8**:1077–89.

47. National Osteoporosis Foundation. *America's Bone Health: The State of Osteoporosis and Low Bone Mass in Our Nation*. Washington, DC: National Osteoporosis Foundation, 2002:1–55.

48. Sanders KM, Nicholson C, Ugoni AM et al. Health burden of hip and other fractures in Australia beyond 2000: Projections based on the Geelong Osteoporosis Study. *Med J Austral* 1999;**170**:467–70.

49. Gullberg B, Johnell O, Kanis JA. World-wide projections for hip fracture. *Osteoporos Int* 1997;**7**: 407–13.

50. Chrischilles E, Shireman T, Wallace R. Costs and health effects of osteoporotic fractures. *Bone* 1994; **15**:377–86.

3

Pathophysiology of osteoporosis

Cyrus Cooper

The key clinical outcome of osteoporosis is fracture, and as outlined in Chapter 2, fractures constitute a major public health problem. This chapter will review the pathophysiology of osteoporosis by considering the structure of bone as a tissue; the function of bone cells (osteoblasts, osteoclasts and osteocytes); and an understanding of the control mechanisms of calcium homeostasis, and the way in which derangements of these lead to osteoporosis.

CHANGES IN BONE MINERAL DENSITY WITH AGING

Peak bone mass

The outline of the skeleton is apparent early in fetal development and the long bones attain their future shape and proportions by about 26 weeks of gestation.[1] From conception to epiphyseal closure, there is a progressive increase in cortical and trabecular bone, which is accelerated during the pre-pubertal growth spurt (Figure 3.1).[2–5] This growth phase produces about 90% of the peak bone mass attained during adult life. The pubertal acceleration of bone gain commences earlier in girls than boys, but by age 20 years the difference in vertebral bone mineral density (BMD) between men and women is slight.[6,7] The precise physiological mechanism of the accelerated bone growth of adolescence is unknown; the spurt in mineral growth parallels the spurt in height, but appears to last longer. In boys, it coincides with a steep rise in serum testosterone concentration, but this is accompanied by a myriad of other endocrinological changes.[8] Following the adolescent growth spurt, BMD undergoes a consolidative phase during which it continues to increase for a 5–15 year period.[9,10] This phase may be critical in determining the overall peak density achieved, as it occurs during a period of many changes in lifestyle.[11]

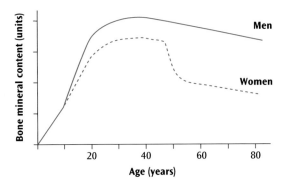

Figure 3.1

Changes in bone mineral with age in men and women.

LOSS OF BONE MINERAL MASS

Skeletal growth and consolidation are followed by a transient period of stability until about the age of 35 years, after which bone loss commences (Figure 3.1).[12] This bone loss is universal[13] in all races and in both sexes, but includes an accelerated phase in the immediate postmenopausal years in women. The differential rates of loss of cortical and trabecular bone, and the varying patterns of loss at different skeletal sites have not been precisely defined. However, there have now been a few published longitudinal studies of bone loss rates at the hip and lumbar spine.[14–16] From these studies in Caucasian ambulatory females in the postmenopause, estimates of loss range from 0.35% to 0.96% loss/year at the femoral neck, 0.32% to 0.95% at the total hip region, 0.3% to 0.75% at the trochanteric region, and 0.36% to 1.14% at the intertrochanteric region. Fewer data are available for men, but a mean annual loss rate of 0.82% at the femoral neck[16] was reported in an Australian cohort aged around 70 years. Over a lifetime, BMD of the femoral neck declines an estimated 58% in women and 39% in men, while BMD of the intertrochanteric region of the proximal femur falls about 53% and 35% in women and men respectively.[17] Estimates of lumbar spine loss rates among women range from 0.39%/year to gains of 0.94%/year; longitudinal studies of men show gains of around 0.5%/year; these 'gains' are artefactual due to osteophytosis.[18] Bone loss is continuous throughout later life, with rates of bone loss increasing at the hip region from 0.32%/year at age 67–69 years to 1.64%/year from age 85 years onwards.[15]

BONE AS A TISSUE

Bone is a metabolically active tissue that is formed, removed and replaced throughout life. Mineralization of its organic matrix produces a tissue of considerable strength and provides the body's store of calcium; this also accounts for the persistence of bone after death and the erroneous impression that it is inert. To understand osteoporosis it is essential to review the structure and physiology of bone, which center around the activity of its specialized cells.[19–26]

The main structural components of bone are the organic matrix, composed predominantly of collagen (a heteropolymeric triple helical molecule arranged in strong fibers), and a mineral (hydroxyapatite), which is laid down upon this matrix in an organized manner by the bone-forming cells, the osteoblasts (Figure 3.2). In the adult skeleton two main anatomical forms of bone are recognized – cortical and trabecular (spongy). The cortical form is composed of tightly packed mineralized bone organized into Haversian systems; these are cylindrical units of compact bone structure built round a central vascular canal and composed of concentric bony lamellae. Cortical bone is largely constructed on the outside shell of the long bones to provide strength on the perimeter of the cylinder. Trabecular bone has a porous sponge-like structure in which trabeculae of bone are joined to each other in the form of a three-dimensional mesh enclosing elements of the bone marrow. This form of bone is found in the vertebral bodies, in particular. The turnover rate of trabecular bone is more rapid than that of cortical bone, owing to its relatively greater surface area; this

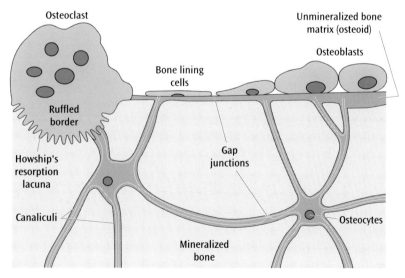

Figure 3.2

Main components of bone.

is one reason why the loss of bone (for instance, after the menopause) is earliest and most rapid in the spine.

COMPONENTS OF BONE

The main components of bone are the organic matrix, bone mineral and bone cells. Organic components of the bone matrix may be divided into collagen and non-collagen protein, as follows:

- Type I collagen (95%)
- Non-collagen substances (5%)
  - proteoglycan
  - osteonectin
  - sialoprotein
  - osteocalcin
  - bone morphogenetic proteins.

There is a large family of genetically different collagens with different structures appropriate to their functions.[27] The most abundant fibrillar collagen and the main collagen of bone is type I.

Collagen is synthesized by the osteoblasts, which are also responsible for its mineralization and which interact with the bone-resorbing cells, the osteoclasts. The osteoblasts are derived from cells of the stromal system, the pre-osteoblasts, and are the precursors of the osteocytes which are found in the mineralized bone. Current evidence suggests that the osteocytes are important as the main route by which mechanical signals induce new bone formation.

BONE MATRIX

Collagen

Collagen, the major extracellular protein in the body, comprises a large family with the common feature of a repetitive Gly-X-Y (gly=glycine, X and Y are often proline and hydroxyproline, respectively) sequence. This molecular structure allows the constituent α-chains to arrange themselves in the form of a triple helix with glycine at its center, and to form intramolecular and inter-molecular crosslinks. The resultant fibers have astonishing tensile strength, provided that the molecular structure (and the subsequent crosslinking) is accurate (Figure 3.3).

Most type I collagen is in the skeleton but it is also found in other tissues, largely on its own (as in tendons and sclerae) and sometimes with other collagens – such as type III in the skin. The relevance of collagen to osteoporosis is as follows:

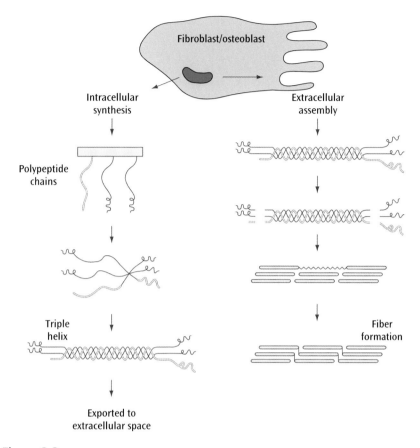

Figure 3.3

The synthesis and structure of type I collagen. The polypeptide chains are synthesized and modified within the cell to form a triple helical molecule that is exported and aggregates into the collagen fiber.

- It contributes to the strength of bone
- Mutations in the genes for type I collagen cause bone fragility (osteogenesis imperfecta)
- It is possible that collagen may sometimes be abnormal in osteoporosis
- Collagen forms a basis for liberalization
- Measurement of its circulating or excreted breakdown products gives an indication of bone turnover and resorption.

Non-collagen proteins

The skeleton contains numerous non-collagen protein constituents, the functions of which are largely unknown; these include the sialoproteins, phosphoproteins and numerous others,[24] including proteoglycans.[28] For many years it has been known that extracts of demineralized bone can induce ectopic ossification, particularly in muscle. The substances that bring this about have now been identified as a family of bone morphogenetic proteins (BMPs).[29] These proteins:

- Are a unique subfamily of transforming growth factor (TGF)β proteins
- Induce ectopic bone
- Influence the pattern of early skeletal development.

The genes for BMPs are related to the large gene family that codes for the TGFβ proteins and also for the proteins concerned with limb patterning and development. These discoveries are of considerable biologic importance as they suggest ways in which the amount of bone within the normal skeleton may be influenced.

BONE MINERAL

There appear to be two different ways in which bone becomes mineralized. In the first, mineral is laid down in association with very small mineralizing vesicles apparently derived from osteoblasts (or chondroblasts). These vesicles contain, and presumably produce, alkaline phosphatase. This enzyme is also a pyrophosphatase and it has been proposed that the breakdown of pyrophosphate (which normally inhibits mineralization) allows mineralization to occur. This system, centered around calcifying vesicles, occurs particularly in the preliminary ossification of cartilage and fetal bone. In mature bone a second mechanism probably predominates. This relies on a template of collagen fibers, which are arranged in a three-dimensional quarter-stagger array that provided regularly alternating gaps or hole zones (Figure 3.3). Observation of experimental systems, such as calcifying turkey tendons, shows the precision of this process. However, despite many suggestions, the exact biochemical basis for mineralization is unknown. It is clear that bone mineral, which is a complex crystalline structure known as hydroxyapatite, adds strength and rigidity to the collagen matrix. In conditions such as rickets and osteomalacia, where mineralization is defective, bone loses its rigidity and is easily deformed. Likewise, where the collagen matrix is faulty, as in osteogenesis imperfecta, the skeleton is excessively fragile.

BONE CELLS

Bone contains specific cells, the osteoblasts, osteoclasts and osteocytes, which are in close association with the bone marrow and the cells of the hemopoietic system.

The osteoblast

The osteoblast is essential for bone formation and lies at the center of bone physiology. It synthesizes bone collagen, non-collagen proteins and alkaline phosphatase and controls mineralization. It also controls the activity of the osteoclasts by mechanisms that are not understood.

The function and behavior of the osteoblasts depend on many factors. These include genetic, mechanical, nutritional and endocrine influences, as well as the effect of local chemical messages produced by the cells – the cytokines.

- Bone mass (and presumably osteoblast function; see also below) is heritable and differs with family, race, collagen gene mutations and possibly changes in the vitamin D receptor
- Mechanical stress stimulates osteoblast function in experimental systems and bone is formed along the lines of stress (Wolff's law), but the mechanisms are unknown. It is possible that osteocytes provide the link that transforms mechanical into biologic systems in bone
- The effects of nutritional endocrine factors on the osteoblast are complex. Although bone size and mass are greater in those who are properly nourished and have a high calcium intake, the reasons for this are not known
- Amongst endocrine factors, the sex hormones and calciotropic hormones are particularly important. Testosterone lack in men and estrogen lack in women reduce bone mass but, again, the mechanisms are not well understood. Osteoblasts contain estrogen receptors, but only a few
- In experimental systems, parathyroid hormone (and some derivatives of it) initially stimulate osteoblast activity. Corticosteroids suppress the activity of the osteoblasts and growth hormone stimulates it
- Finally, the osteoblast appears to act as an intermediate between various hormone systems and the osteoclast.

The osteoclast

The osteoclast is a multinucleated cell derived from precursors within the hemopoietic system. It is a specialized bone-resorbing cell that seals off an area of the bone surface to produce a very acid environment within which its lysosomal enzymes resorb whole bone. The hydrogen ions necessary for this activity are produced by the carbonic anhydrase system (Figure 3.4). Absence of this enzyme causes a rare form of osteopetrosis (marble bone disease) because bone resorption is defective; other defects of osteoclast function may lead to osteopetrosis in humans and animals. Calcitonin directly suppresses the osteoclast. Current evidence suggests that the effects of other hormones, such as parathyroid hormone, which increase bone resorption, are mediated via the osteoblast.

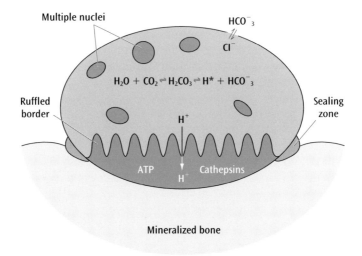

Figure 3.4

Important features of the osteoclast. Resorption occurs within the acid sealed zone.

The osteocyte

The osteocyte, derived from the osteoblast, lies within mineralized bone and communicates with its neighbors through its extensions in the canaliculi. This cell may detect mechanical deformation and mediate the osteoblast response to this.

Bone multicellular units

The skeleton is constantly being resorbed and rebuilt by teams of bone cells. In youth, these processes favor synthesis; in old age they favor resorption. The cellular system around which this balance is centered is the bone multi-cellular unit (BMU; also known as the bone remodeling unit, BRU). There are innumerable BMUs on the surface of trabecular bone and within the cortex, which are at different stages in their life cycle. This cycle begins with the activation of bone resorption and ends with the replacement of bone by osteoblasts (Figure 3.5). These cycles may each take up to 6 months (Figure 3.6). The possible therapeutic manipulation of BMUs is important in considering how bone loss may be prevented or bone mass increased. This is likely to be more effective in the young skeleton than in the old, because of the larger number of active BMUs in youth.

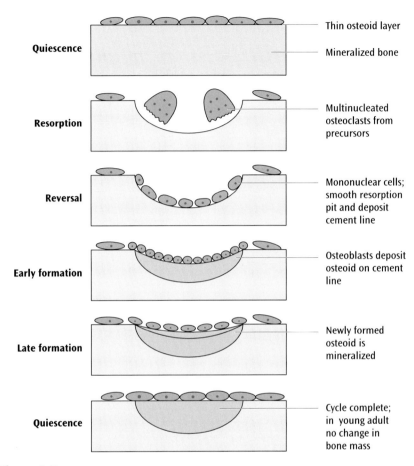

Figure 3.5

Changes that occur in the bone multicellular unit (BMU). This represents the surface of trabecular bone; similar changes occur in the cortical bone.

Bone cell conversation

There is good evidence to suggest that the activities of the osteoblasts and osteoclasts are normally closely linked under physiological and pathological conditions (for instance in Paget's disease) but the mechanisms for the linkage are not understood. Bone cells (and other cells) produce a great variety of locally acting cell-derived substances called cytokines, which can be shown to have many different actions in experimental systems.

The major cytokines comprise:

- Interleukins
- Tumor necrosis factors

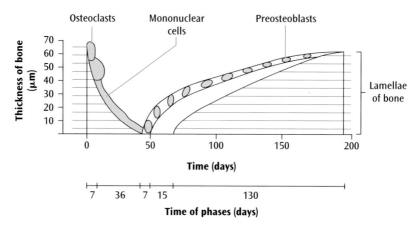

Figure 3.6

Estimated time-scale of a bone-remodeling cycle.

- Interferons
- Growth factors
- Colony-stimulating factors.

The physiological function of the cytokines is largely unknown.[25,30]

One particular problem is how the BMU cycle begins. There is some evidence that the osteoblast produces osteoclast-activating factors (OAFs); there is also some evidence that the resorption of bone may release biologically active bone mitogenic substances that turn on osteoblastic activity.

CALCIUM AND PHOSPHATE BALANCE

The central position of calcium as an ionic messenger continues to be explored. It is essential for innumerable functions such as reproduction, neurotransmission, hormone action, cellular growth and enzyme action. There have been considerable advances in our understanding of the messengers that control cellular processes by generating internal calcium signals. Chief amongst these is inositol triphosphate, which is generated via G-protein and tyrosine kinase-linked receptors.

Much is now known about external calcium balance and the main hormones that control it; phosphate balance is less well understood. The circulating concentration of plasma calcium is determined by the amount of calcium absorbed by the intestine, the amount excreted by the kidney, and the exchange of mineral with the skeleton. The relative importance of these exchanges differs during growth and pregnancy and in different disorders. Total plasma calcium is closely maintained between 2.25 mmol/l and 2.60 mmol/l, of which nearly half is in the ionized form (47% ionized, 46% protein bound, and the remainder complexed). The skeleton contains approximately 1 kg (25,000 mmol) of calcium.

Parathyroid hormone

The gene for parathyroid hormone (PTH) is on chromosome 11. The hormone is synthesized as a large precursor like other proteins packaged for export. Its secretion is stimulated by a reduction in the plasma concentration of ionized calcium. Parathyroid cells respond to changes in the extracellular concentration of calcium via a recently identified calcium-sensing receptor.

An increase in PTH leads to an increase in calcium absorption through the gut, in calcium reabsorption through the kidney, and in bone resorption. Intestinal calcium absorption is mediated by the active metabolite of vitamin D, 1,25-dihydroxycholecalciferol (1,25-$(OH)_2D_3$). In contrast, the effect of parathyroid hormone on renal calcium reabsorption is direct. The cellular effects of PTH on kidney and bone appear to utilize more than one system. PTH encourages osteoclastic bone resorption by its effects on the osteoblast, as previously described.

Vitamin D

Vitamin D is synthesized either as vitamin D_3 (cholecalciferol) within the skin from its precursor 7-dehydrocholesterol under the influence of ultraviolet light (usually as sunlight), or taken in with food, either as vitamin D_3 or D_2 (ergocalciferol). It is subsequently transported to the liver by a binding protein where it undergoes 25-hydroxylation; 25-hydroxyvitamin D (25(OH)D) is then hydroxylated in the 1 position by the renal 1α-hydroxylase. The classic action of the active metabolite, 1,25$(OH)_2D$, is on calcium metabolism, promoting the synthesis of a calcium-transporting protein within the cells of the small intestine. Its effects are mediated through a widely distributed vitamin D receptor with DNA and hormone-binding components.[31] It is now known that 1,25$(OH)_2D$ has many effects outside mineral metabolism, concerned with the immune system and the growth and differentiation of a wide variety of cells.

Measurement of plasma 25(OH)D has proved to be a useful indicator of vitamin D status, and work on 1,25$(OH)_2D$ and its receptors has identified the causes of the rarer forms of inherited rickets. Although the kidney is the main source of 1,25$(OH)_2D$, this metabolite can also be synthesized by a variety of granulomata, which provides a partial explanation for the hypercalcemia of sarcoidosis and (occasionally) lymphomas. Some, but not all work suggests that bone mass is partly linked to certain polymorphic changes in the vitamin D receptor gene.[32]

Calcitonin

The main effect of administered calcitonin is to reduce bone resorption by direct and reversible suppression of the osteoclast. The physiological role of calcitonin is uncertain, although it is thought to protect the skeleton during such stresses as growth and pregnancy.

Parathyroid hormone-related protein

The hormone parathyroid hormone-related protein (PTHrP) was discovered during studies on patients with non-metastatic hypercalcemia of malignancy. It has close sequence homology with PTH at the amino-terminal end of the molecule and has very similar effects. Its gene is on the short arm of chromosome 12, thought to have arisen by a duplication of chromosome 11, which carries the human PTH gene. It has been detected in a number of tumors, particularly of the lung. There is also evidence that it may have a role in fetal physiology, controlling the calcium gradient across the placenta and maintaining the relatively higher concentrations in the fetal circulation, and in cartilage development.

Other hormones

Apart from the recognized calciotropic hormones, the skeleton is influenced by corticosteroids, the sex hormones, thyroxine, and growth hormone, as follows:

- Excess corticosteroids (either therapeutic or in Cushing's disease) are associated with increased bone resorption, reduced bone formation and altered microarchitecture
- Both androgens and estrogens promote and maintain skeletal mass, osteoblasts have receptors for estrogens, although they are not abundant
- Thyroxine increases bone turnover and increases resorption in excess of formation; thyrotoxicosis thus reduces bone mass
- Excess growth hormone leads to gigantism and acromegaly (according to the age of onset) with enlargement of the bones; absence of growth hormone will lead to proportional short stature; where there is wider pituitary failure, the reduction in gonadotrophins will cause bone loss.

BIOCHEMICAL MEASUREMENTS OF BONE CELL ACTIVITY

Knowledge of bone physiology enables biochemical measures of bone turnover to be interpreted. Such measures include the plasma bone-derived alkaline phosphatase and osteocalcin, and urinary total hydroxyproline and crosslinked collagen-derived peptides. The first two of these are closely related to osteoblast function, and the second two to bone resorption. As formation and resorption are closely coupled, such measurements are usually also closely related to each other, and to overall bone turnover.

Plasma alkaline phosphatase (largely derived from osteoblasts) provides a reliable and readily accessible index of bone formation, being increased during periods of rapid growth and particularly where bone turnover is greatly increased, as in Paget's disease; where more skeletal specificity is required, measurement of bone-derived (rather than total) alkaline phosphatase can be useful.

- Early measurements of serum osteocalcin (bone Gla protein) were widely variable and depended on the origin, sensitivity and stability of the antibodies used
- Total urine hydroxyproline is influenced by dietary collagen (gelatin) and reflects both resorption and new collagen synthesis
- The recent development of methods for the measurement of urinary collagen-derived pyridinium crosslinks promises to give a reliable indication of bone resorption unrelated to new collagen formation and not influenced by diet.[33] This may be particularly useful in detecting the suppression of bone resorption by the newly available anti-resorptive bisphosphonates, such as alendronate (see Chapter 5)
- Other research methods include measurement of circulating fragments of the collagen molecule derived from its carboxy-terminal and amino-terminal extensions which, under certain circumstances, indicate the rate of collagen (bone) formation.

CONCLUSIONS

Bone is a metabolically active tissue composed of mineralized organic bone matrix produced by specialized bone cells. These cells work in teams to remove (osteoclasts) and to replace (osteoblasts) bone tissue. Changes in bone mass depend on the balance between these activities. The strength of bone depends on its structure (cortical or trabecular), and on the integrity of its mineral (hydroxyapatite) and matrix (collagen) components. The activity of bone cells can be assessed by biochemical measurement. The amount of bone and its density varies with age and disease. The main determinants of bone mass include the genetic and early environmental influences that determine peak bone mass and a series of factors which are predisposed to accelerated bone loss (estrogen deficiency, low body mass index, cigarette smoking, alcohol consumption, physical inactivity and reduced dietary calcium intake). These individual risk factors are important in determining risk-based strategies to prevent osteoporotic fracture.

REFERENCES

1. Cooper C. Bone mass throughout life: bone growth and involution. In: Francis R, ed. *Osteoporosis: Pathogenesis and Management*. London: Kluwer, 1990:1–26.

2. Mazess RB, Cameron JR. Growth of bone in school children: comparison of radiographic morphometry and photon absorptiometry. *Growth* 1972; **36**:77–92.

3. Landin L, Nilsson BE. Forearm bone mineral content in children. Normative data. *Acta Paediatr Scand* 1981;**70**: 919–23.

4. Riggs BL, Wahner HW, Melton LJ, Richelson LS, Judd HL, Offord KP. Rates of bone loss in the appendicular and axial skeletons of women. Evidence of substantial vertebral bone loss before menopause. *J Clin Invest* 1986;**77**:1487–91.

5. Specker BL, Brazerol W, Tsang RC, Levin R, Searcy J, Steichen J. Bone mineral content in children 1 to 6 years of age. Detectable sex differences after 4 years of age. *Am J Dis Child* 1987;**141**:343–4.

6. Kelly PJ, Eisman JA, Sambrook PN. Interaction of genetic and environmental influences on peak bone density. *Osteoporos Int* 1990;**1**:56–60.

7. Kelly PJ, Twomey L, Sambrook PN, Eisman JA. Sex differences in peak adult bone mineral density. *J Bone Miner Res* 1990;**5**:1169–75.

8. Krabbe S, Christiansen C, Rodbro P, Transbol I. Effect of puberty on rates of bone growth and mineralisation: with observations in male delayed puberty. *Arch Dis Child* 1979;**54**: 950–3.

9. Kleerekoper M, Tolia K, Parfitt AM. Nutritional, endocrine, and demographic aspects of osteoporosis. *Orthop Clin North Am* 1981;**12**: 547–58.

10. Recker RR, Davies KM, Hinders SM, Heaney RP, Stegman MR, Kimmel DB. Bone gain in young adult women. *JAMA* 1992;**268**:2403–8.

11. Slemenda C, Johnston CC, Hui SL. Patterns of bone loss and physiologic growing. In: *Proceedings of the Third International Symposium on Osteoporosis*. Copenhagen: Osteoporosis ApS, 1990:99.

12. Cooper C. Epidemiological aspects of osteoporosis and age-related fractures. In: Ring EFJ, Evans WD, Dixon AS, eds. *Osteoporosis and Bone Mineral Measurement*. York, UK: IPSM publications, 1989.

13. Garn SM, Rohmann CG, Wagner B. Bone loss as a general phenomenon in man. *Fed Proc* 1967;**26**:1729–36.

14. Dennison E, Eastell R, Fall CHD, Kellingray S, Wood PJ, Cooper C. Determinants of bone loss in elderly men and women: A prospective population-based study. *Osteoporos Int* 1999;**10**:384–39.

15. Ensrud KE, Palermo L, Black DM et al. Hip and calcaneal bone loss increase with advancing age: longitudinal results from the study of osteoporotic fractures. *J Bone Miner Res* 1995;**10**: 1778–87.

16. Jones G, Nguyen T, Sambrook P, Kelly PJ, Eisman JA. Progressive loss of bone in the femoral neck in elderly people: longitudinal findings from the Dubbo osteoporosis epidemiology study. *BMJ* 1994;**309**:691–5.

17. Cooper C, Melton LJ. Magnitude and impact of osteoporosis and fractures. In: Marcus R. Feldman D, Kelsey J, eds. *Osteoporosis*, Vol 2, 2nd edn. San Diego: Academic Press, 1996:419–34.

18. Slemenda CW, Christian JC, Reed T, Reister TK, Williams CJ, Johnston CC Jr. Long-term bone loss in men: effects of genetic and environmental factors. *Ann Intern Med* 1992;**117**:286–91.

19. Smith R. Bone in health and disease. In: Maddison PJ, Isenberg DA, Woo P, Glass DN, eds. *Oxford Textbook of Rheumatology* 2nd edn. Oxford University Press, 1997:421–40.

20. Noda M. *Cellular and Molecular Biology of Bone*. San Diego: Academic Press, 1993.

21. Raisz LG. Physiology of bone. In: Becker KI, ed. *Principles and Practice of Endocrinology and Metabolism,* 2nd edn. Philadelphia: Lippincott 1995: 447–55.

22. Royce PM, Steinmann B. *Connective Tissue and its Heritable Disorders.* New York: Wiley-Liss, 1993.

23. Marcus R, Feldman D, Kelsey J. *Osteoporosis* Vol 2, 2nd edn. New York: Academic Press, 1996.

24. Bilézikian JP, Raisz LG, Rodan GA. *Principles of Bone Biology.* San Diego; Academic Press, 1996.

25. Macdonald BR, Gowen M. The cell biology of bone. *Baillière's Clinical Rheumatology.* 1993;**7**:421–43.

26. Smith R. Disorders of the skeleton. In: Weatherall DJ, Ledingham JGG, Warrell DA, eds. *Oxford Textbook of Medicine,* 3rd edn. Oxford University Press, 1995: 3055–95.

27. Hulmes DJS. The collagen super family – diverse structures and assemblies. *Essays Biochem* 1992;**27**:49–67.

28. Hardingham TE, Fosang AJ. Proteoglycans: many forms and many functions. *FASEB J* 1992;**6**:861–70.

29. Wozney JM. Bone morphogenetic proteins and their gene expression. In: Noda N, ed. *Cellular and Molecular Biology of Bone.* New York: Academic Press, 1993:131–67.

30. Manolagas SC, Jilka RL. Bone marrow, cytokines and bone remodelling. *N Eng J Med* 1995;**332**:305–11.

31. Fraser DR. Vitamin D. *Lancet* 1995; **345**:104–6.

32. Spector TD, Keen RW, Arden NK et al. Influence of vitamin D receptor genotype on bone mineral density in postmenopausal women; a twin study in Britain. *BMJ* 1995;**310**:1357–60.

33. Editorial. Pyridinium cross links as markers of bone resorption. *Lancet* 1992;**240**:278–9.

4
Risk stratification

John A Kanis

INTRODUCTION

The increasing prevalence and awareness of osteoporosis, together with the development of treatments of proven efficacy, will increase the demand for management of patients with osteoporosis. This in turn will require widespread facilities for the assessment of osteoporosis. Measurements of bone mineral are a central component of any provision which arises from the internationally agreed description of osteoporosis: a systemic disease characterized by low bone mass and micro-architectural deterioration of bone tissue, with a consequent increase in bone fragility and susceptibility to fracture.[1] The diagnosis thus centers on the assessment of bone mass and quality. There are no satisfactory clinical tools available to assess bone quality independently of bone density, so that for practical purposes the diagnosis of osteoporosis depends upon the measurement of skeletal mass, as assessed by measurements of bone mineral density (BMD).

The clinical significance of osteoporosis is the fractures that arise with their attendant morbidity and mortality. Although bone mass is an important component of the risk of fracture, other abnormalities occur in the skeleton that contribute to fragility. In addition, a variety of non-skeletal factors, such as the liability to fall and force of impact, contribute to fracture risk. Since BMD forms but one component of fracture risk, accurate assessment of fracture risk should ideally take into account other readily measured indices of fracture risk that add information to that provided by BMD.

The identification of risk factors for fracture has been widely used in case finding strategies. In such schemes, patients are identified on the basis of clinical risk factors. Examples include a family history of fragility fracture, a previous fragility fracture, low body mass index and the long-term use of corticosteroids. Patients so identified are referred for BMD measurements, and intervention offered if BMD falls below a given threshold. Current guidelines in Europe suggest that intervention should be offered in those individuals subsequently shown to have osteoporosis (i.e. a T-score of −2.5 SD or less).[2,3] In the USA a less stringent threshold is recommended of −2.0 SD in the absence of significant risk factors, and −1.5 SD in the presence of risk factors.[4] This case finding strategy is conservative. Individuals must have one of the chosen risk factors before they are referred for BMD under the current guidance of the International Osteoporosis Foundation (IOF). Moreover, the vast majority of fractures will occur in those individuals who are never assessed. Against this background a growing view is that the assessment of fracture risk should encompass all aspects of risk and that intervention should not be guided solely on the basis of BMD.[5,6] There is a distinction to be made, therefore, between diagnosis of osteoporosis and the assessment of fracture risk, that in turn implies a distinction between diagnostic and intervention thresholds. This chapter reviews the extent that this can be achieved in clinical practice.

DIAGNOSIS OF OSTEOPOROSIS

The cornerstone for the diagnosis of osteoporosis lies in the assessment of BMD. In 1994, an expert panel of the World Health Organization (WHO) recommended thresholds of BMD in women to define osteoporosis[7,8] that have been widely, but not universally, accepted by the international scientific community and by regulatory agencies.[9–11] Osteoporosis in postmenopausal Caucasian women is defined as a value for BMD more than 2.5 SD below the young adult average value. Severe osteoporosis (established osteoporosis) uses the same threshold, but in the presence of one or more fragility fracture. The preferred site for diagnostic purposes are BMD measurements made at the hip, either at the total hip or the femoral neck.[5] For men, the same threshold as utilized for women is appropriate since for any given BMD, the age-adjusted fracture risk is more or less the same.[12–15]

The diagnostic threshold identifies approximately 16% of postmenopausal women as having osteoporosis when measurements using dual-energy X-ray absorptiometry (DXA) are made at the hip.[7,8] Table 4.1 displays the proportion of white women with osteoporosis by age group in the USA.

The diagnostic use of the T-score cannot be used interchangeably with different techniques and at different sites, since the same T-score derived from different sites and techniques yields different information on fracture risk.[16] For example, in women aged 60, the average T-score ranges from −0.7 SD to −2.5 SD, depending on the technique used. Reasons include differences in the gradient of risk for techniques to predict fracture, differences in the population standard deviation, and differences in the apparent rates of bone loss with age. A further problem is that inter-site correlations, although usually of statistical significance, are inadequate for predictive purposes in individuals giving rise to errors of mis-classification.[17] This does not mean that other sites and other techniques cannot be used for risk assessment; only that the performance characteristics of the different techniques differ.

Table 4.1   Proportion (%) of white women with osteoporosis by age adjusted to 1990 US white women defined as a bone mass below 2.5 SD of the young adult reference range at the hip, spine or forearm[7,8]

Age range (years)	Any site*	Hip alone
50–59	14.8	3.9
60–69	21.6	8.0
70–79	38.5	24.5
80+	70.0	47.5
≥50	30.3	16.2

*Hip, spine or forearm.

ASSESSMENT OF FRACTURE RISK

The use of bone mass measurements for prognosis depends upon accuracy. Accuracy in this context is the ability of the measurement to predict fracture. In general, all absorptiometric techniques have high specificity but low sensitivity which vary with the cut-off chosen to designate high risk. Many cross-sectional prospective population studies indicate that the risk for fracture increases by a factor of 1.5 to 3.0 for each standard deviation decrease in BMD as summarized in Table 4.2.[18] Accuracy is improved by site-specific measurements (see Table 4.2), so that for forearm fractures, the risk might ideally be measured at the forearm, and for hip fracture, measurements made at the hip. In the immediate postmenopausal population, measurements at any site (hip, spine and wrist) predict any osteoporotic fracture equally well with a gradient of risk of approximately 1.5 per standard deviation decrease in BMD.

Table 4.2   Age-adjusted relative increase in risk of fracture (with 95% confidence interval) in women for every 1 SD decrease in bone mineral density (absorptiometry) below the mean value for age[18]

Site of measurement	Forearm fracture	Hip fracture	Vertebral fracture	All fractures
Distal radius	1.7 (1.4–2.0)	1.8 (1.4–2.2)	1.7 (1.4–2.1)	1.4 (1.3–1.6)
Femoral neck	1.4 (1.4–1.6)	2.6 (2.0–3.5)	1.8 (1.1–2.7)	1.6 (1.4–1.8)
Lumbar spine	1.5 (1.3–1.8)	1.6 (1.2–2.2)	2.3 (1.9–2.8)	1.5 (1.4–1.7)

The highest gradient of risk is found at the hip to predict hip fracture where the gradient of risk is 2.6. Thus, an individual with a T-score of −3 SD at the hip would have a 2.6^3 or greater than 15-fold higher risk than an individual with a BMD at the mean for young adults. By contrast, the same T-score at the spine would yield a much lower risk estimate – an approximate 4-fold increase (1.6^3).

Despite these performance characteristics, it should be recognized that, just because BMD is normal, there is no guarantee that a fracture will not occur – only that the risk is decreased. Conversely, if BMD is in the osteoporotic range, then fractures are more likely, but not invariable. At the age of 50 years, the proportion of women with osteoporosis who will fracture their hip, spine or forearm or proximal humerus in the next 10 years (i.e. positive predictive value) is approximately 45%. The detection rate for these fractures (sensitivity) is, however, low and 96% of such fractures would occur in women without osteoporosis.[19] The low sensitivity is one of the reasons why widespread population-based screening is not recommended in women at the time of the menopause.

Fracture risk is commonly expressed as a relative risk, as the risk in individuals with a risk factor compared to the risk in those without the factor. However, it is also important to consider the absolute risk of fracture. This depends upon age and life expectancy as well as the current relative risk. In general, remaining lifetime risk of fracture increases with age up to the age of 70 years or so. Thereafter, probability plateaus and then decreases since the risk of death with age outstrips the increasing evidence of fracture with age. Estimates of lifetime risk are of value in considering the burden of osteoporosis in the community, and the effects of intervention strategies. For several reasons they are less relevant for assessing risk of individuals in whom treatment might be envisaged. First, treatments are not presently given for a lifetime, due variably to side effects of continued treatment (e.g. hormone replacement therapy) or low continuance (most treatments). Moreover, the feasibility of life-long interventions has never been tested, either using high risk or global strategies. Second, the predictive value of low BMD and some other risk factors for fracture risk is attenuated over time.[20] Finally, the confidence in estimates decreases with time due to the uncertainties concerning future mortality trends.[21] For this reason, the IOF and the WHO recommend that risk of fracture should be expressed as a short-term absolute risk (i.e. probability over a 10 year interval).[6] The period of 10 years covers the likely duration of treatment and the benefits that may continue once treatment is stopped.

A further advantage of utilizing absolute fracture probability in risk assessment, is that it standardizes the output from the multiple techniques and sites used for assessment. The estimated probability will of course depend upon the performance characteristics (gradient of risk) provided by any technique at any one site. Moreover, it also permits the presence or absence of risk factors other than BMD to be computed as a single metric. This is important because there are many risk factors that give information over and above that provided by BMD. The most important of these is age.

AGE AND BONE MINERAL DENSITY

The same T-score with the same technique at any one site has a different significance at different ages. Fracture risk is much higher in the elderly than in the young.[22] This is because age contributes to risk independently of BMD. Indeed, from knowledge of the relationship between BMD and fracture risk it would be predicted that fracture risk might increase 4-fold between the ages of 50 and 80 years. In reality for hip fracture the risk increases 30-fold, indicating that over a lifetime, changes in age have an approximately 7-fold greater effect than changes in BMD. It also indicates the independent value of assessing age.

The relationship between age, BMD and fracture probability at the spine and hip is given in Tables 4.3 and 4.4.[23] At the threshold for osteoporosis (T-score = −2.5 SD), the probability of hip fracture ranges from 10.5% to 1.4% in men and women, respectively (see Table 4.3).[23] Any difference in probability between men and women is not marked since the same BMD carries a similar risk in both sexes. The relationship between T-score and spine fracture probability is shown in Table 4.4.[23] At any given T-score there is approximately a 2- to 3-fold increase in probability with age between the ages of 50 and 85

Table 4.3 Ten year probability of hip fracture in Swedish men and women according to age and BMD at the femoral neck[23]

Age (years)	Population	T-score −1	T-score −2.5	T-score ≤2.5
Men				
45	0.5	0.7	2.2	3.4
50	0.8	1.1	3.4	5.1
55	0.8	0.9	3.1	4.9
60	1.2	1.2	3.7	6.0
65	2.1	1.9	5.3	8.8
70	3.4	2.7	8.5	14.3
75	5.9	4.1	14.2	24.2
80	7.6	4.6	13.7	24.3
85	7.1	7.6	10.5	19.9
Women				
45	0.4	0.4	1.4	2.2
50	0.6	0.5	1.7	2.9
55	1.2	0.7	2.9	4.9
60	2.3	1.1	4.4	7.8
65	3.9	1.5	5.9	11.3
70	7.3	2.0	8.8	18.3
75	11.7	2.3	11.1	24.6
80	15.5	2.5	11.5	27.9
85	16.1	2.1	10.0	25.8

Table 4.4 Ten year probability of clinically apparent spine fracture in Swedish men and women by age and T-score at the femoral neck[23]

Age (years)	T-score					
	0	−1	−2.0	−2.5	−3.0	−4.0
Men						
50	0.9	1.5	2.5	3.2	4.1	6.9
55	1.0	1.7	2.9	3.8	5.0	8.5
60	1.1	1.9	3.1	3.9	5.0	8.1
65	1.4	2.2	3.4	4.2	5.3	8.3
70	1.8	2.9	4.7	6.0	7.6	12.2
75	1.9	3.3	5.6	7.2	9.4	15.6
80	2.1	3.4	5.5	6.9	8.7	13.7
85	1.9	2.9	4.4	5.4	6.7	10.1
Women						
50	0.6	1.1	2.0	2.6	3.5	6.1
55	0.7	1.4	2.5	3.4	4.6	8.3
60	1.0	1.9	3.4	4.6	6.1	11.0
65	1.4	2.6	4.7	6.2	8.3	14.6
70	1.6	2.9	5.5	7.4	10.0	18.0
75	1.3	2.5	5.0	6.9	9.5	17.9
80	1.2	2.4	4.6	6.3	8.7	16.1
85	1.1	2.1	4.0	5.5	7.5	13.6

years. For any given age there is approximately a 4- to 5-fold increase in probability between a T-score of 0 and −2.5 SD. Thus, the consideration of age and BMD together increases the range of risk that can be identified. Imagine, for the sake of argument, that one wished to treat individuals with a greater than 10% probability of spine fracture, then very few individuals would be identified at the age of 50 years on the basis of BMD. The addition of age as a risk factor would, however, identify a substantial minority of individuals above this threshold risk.

OTHER RISK FACTORS

A large number of additional risk factors for fracture have been identified, as seen in Table 4.5.[24] For the purposes of risk assessment interest lies in those factors that contribute significantly to fracture risk over and above that provided by BMD measurements or age. Thus, the presence of multiple risk factors can be used to enhance a case finding strategy in osteoporosis by increasing the dynamic range of risk stratification. Several caveats apply. Some risk factors vary in importance according to age. For example, risk factors for

Table 4.5 Risks for osteoporotic fractures[24]	
Female gender	Premature menopause
Age*	Primary or secondary amenorrhoea Primary and secondary hypogonadism in man
Asian or Caucasian race	Previous fragility fracture*
Low BMD	Glucocorticoid therapy*
High bone turnover*	Family history of hip fracture*
Poor visual acuity*	Low body weight*
Neuromuscular disorders*	Cigarette smoking* Excessive alcohol consumption* Prolonged immobilization Low dietary calcium intake Vitamin D deficiency

*These characteristics capture aspects of fracture risk over and above that provided by BMD.

falling, such as visual impairment, reduced mobility and treatment with sedatives, are more strongly predictive of fracture in the elderly than in younger individuals.[25] Some risk factors are not amenable to pharmacologic treatments, so that the relationship between absolute probability of fracture and reversible risk is important. Liability to falls is an appropriate example where the risk of fracture is high, but treatment with agents affecting bone metabolism may have little effect on risk. Other risk factors, such as prior fragility fractures, contribute to a risk that is responsive to intervention.

Glucocorticoids are an important cause of osteoporosis and fractures.[26,27] Bone loss is believed to be most rapid in the first few months of treatment, and affects both axial and appendicular sites. Loss is most marked at the spine where cancellous bone predominates. The fracture risk conferred by the use of corticosteroids is, however, not solely dependent upon bone loss and BMD-independent risks have been identified.[28] In a recent meta-analysis the relative risk (RR) of hip fracture was increased 2.1- to 4.4-fold, depending upon age.[27] Table 4.6 displays these results.

Many studies indicate that history of fragility fracture is an important risk factor for further fracture.[29] Fracture risk is approximately doubled in the presence of a prior fracture. The increase in risk is even more marked for a vertebral fracture following a previous spine fracture. For example, the presence of two or more prevalent vertebral fractures was associated with a 12-fold increase in fracture risk for any given BMD.[30] A recent meta-analysis showing risks according to the site of a prior fracture is given in Table 4.7.[29]

Table 4.6 Risk of hip fracture associated with ever-use of corticosteroids compared with never-use according to age, with and without adjustment for BMD[28]

Age (years)	Without BMD		With BMD	
	RR	95% CI	RR	95% CI
50	3.47	0.99–12.21	4.42	1.26–15.49
55	3.47	1.25–9.60	4.15	1.50–11.49
60	3.26	1.47–7.24	3.71	1.67–8.23
65	2.69	1.40–5.16	2.98	1.55–5.74
70	2.22	1.26–3.91	2.44	1.37–4.36
75	2.16	1.37–3.41	2.22	1.35–3.63
80	2.25	1.53–3.30	2.13	1.39–3.27
85	2.42	1.59–3.67	2.48	1.58–3.89

Table 4.7 Meta-analysis of the risk of fracture in women with a prior fracture at the sites shown[29]

Site of prior fracture	Risk of subsequent fracture at:			
	Hip	Spine	Forearm	Minor fracture
Hip	2.3	2.5	1.4	1.9
Spine	2.3	4.4	1.4	1.8
Forearm	1.9	1.7	3.3	2.4
Minor fracture	2.0	1.9	1.8	1.9

BIOCHEMICAL ASSESSMENT OF FRACTURE RISK

Bone markers are increased after the menopause, and in several studies the rate of bone loss varies according to the marker value.[31] Thus, a potential clinical application of biochemical indices of skeletal metabolism is in assessing fracture risk. Prospective studies have shown an association of osteoporotic fracture with indices of bone turnover independent of BMD in women at the time of the menopause and in elderly women.[32–34] In elderly women with values for resorption markers exceeding the reference range for premenopausal women, fracture risk is increased approximately 2-fold after adjusting for BMD. These studies suggest that a combined approach using BMD with indices of bone turnover may improve fracture prediction in postmenopausal women.[35]

INTEGRATING RISK FACTORS

How can the combined intelligence of the presence or absence of risk factors, BMD and age be factored into estimates of fracture probability? The general relationship between relative risk and 10 year probability of hip fracture is shown in Table 4.8.[19] For example, a woman at the age of 60 has, on average, a 10 year probability of hip fracture of 2.4% (see Table 4.8). In the presence of a prior fragility fracture this risk is increased approximately 2-fold and the probability increases to 4.8%. The integration of risk factors is not new and has been successfully applied in the management of coronary heart disease.[36]

There are, however, a number of problems to be resolved before all BMD-independent risk factors can be utilized. Although corticosteroid treatment confers a risk over and above that afforded by age and BMD, as does a prior fragility fracture, the relationship between corticosteroid use and prior fragility fracture has not yet been explored. Until these interrelationships are established and validated on an international basis, the integration of multiple risk factors must be used cautiously.

Table 4.8   Ten-year probability of fracture in men and women from Sweden according to age and the relative risk (RR) to the average population[19]

	Age (years)			
RR	50	60	70	80
Hip fracture				
Men				
1	0.84	1.26	3.68	9.53
2	1.68	2.50	7.21	17.89
3	2.51	3.73	10.59	25.26
4	3.33	4.94	13.83	31.75
Women				
1	0.57	2.40	7.87	18.00
2	1.14	4.75	15.10	32.0
3	1.71	7.04	21.70	42.9
4	2.27	9.27	27.70	51.6
Hip, clinical spine, humeral or Colles' fracture				
Men				
1	3.3	4.7	7.0	12.6
2	6.5	9.1	13.5	23.1
3	9.6	13.3	19.4	13.9
4	12.6	17.3	24.9	39.3
Women				
1	5.8	9.6	16.1	21.5
2	11.3	18.2	29.4	37.4
3	16.5	26.0	40.0	49.2
4	21.4	33.1	49.5	58.1

OPTIMIZATION OF CASE FINDING STRATEGY

It is evident that the consideration of multiple risk factors improves risk strat-ification of individuals so that those above a given threshold can be offered treatment. The interrelationship between BMD, age and other independent risk factors is now established, although the relationship between the clinical risk factors has yet to be formalized.

The question arises whether a BMD test is required in all individuals who are offered treatment. The value of pharmacologic agents in decreasing fracture risk has been best quantified in those identified on the basis of low BMD. Indeed, for some interventions, treatment of individuals without osteoporosis may yield less in terms of fracture dividends but in other studies individuals with osteopenia respond to treatment with the same relative risk reduction. In this regard the question arises whether patients identified on the basis of clin-ical risk factors alone have a risk identified that would be amenable to thera-peutic manipulation. Although risk factors, such as a prior fragility fracture, are 'independent' of BMD they are not totally independent in the sense that patients identified on the basis of fragility fracture do have low BMD. Moreover, patients selected only on the basis of fracture have been shown to respond to therapeutic intervention with bisphosphonates. Thus, individuals selected on the basis of clinical risk factors are likely to have a low BMD. If this assumption is accepted, then the following strategy can be envisaged. The first step is an assessment of fracture probability that is based solely on clinical risk factors. This is expected to identify three groups of individuals.

The first are those at very high risk above an intervention threshold in whom a BMD test would not alter their classification. These patients can be offered treatment irrespective of BMD. In practice BMD might be measured so that response to treatment can be monitored.

A second group comprises individuals who, on the basis of clinical risk factor assessment, have a very low probability of osteoporotic fracture, so low that the estimate of BMD would not alter their stratification to be above a given level of risk.

An intermediate group are those in whom fracture probability is close to an intervention threshold where the probability is higher that a BMD test might re-categorize individuals at high to low risk (or vice versa). The formalization of this approach is not yet complete, but preliminary evidence from a variety of prospectively studied cohorts suggests that a minority of individuals would require a BMD test on this basis.

CONCLUSIONS

The diagnosis of osteoporosis centers on the assessment of BMD at the hip using DXA. However, other sites and validated techniques can be used for frac-ture prediction. Several clinical risk factors contribute to fracture risk independently of BMD. These include age, prior fragility fracture, premature menopause, a family history of hip fracture and the use of oral corticosteroids. The use of these risk factors in conjunction with BMD improves sensitivity of fracture prediction.

In the absence of validated population screening strategies, a case finding strategy is recommended based on the assessment of fracture probability utilizing clinical risk factors and where appropriate additional testing, such as BMD. With the multiple techniques available for fracture risk assessment, and the multiple fracture outcomes, the desirable measurement to determine intervention thresholds is 10 year probability of fracture.

REFERENCES

1. Anonymous. Consensus development conference: Diagnosis, prophylaxis and treatment of osteoporosis. *Am J Med* 1993;**94**:646–50.

2. Kanis JA, Delmas P, Burckhardt P, Cooper C, Torgerson D, on behalf of the European Foundation for Osteoporosis and Bone Disease. Guidelines for diagnosis and management of osteoporosis. *Osteoporosis Int* 1997;**7**:390–406.

3. Royal College of Physicians. *Clinical Guidelines for the Prevention and Treatment of Osteoporosis*. London: RCP, 1999.

4. National Osteoporosis Foundation. Analyses of the effectiveness and cost of screening and treatment strategies for osteoporosis: a basis for development of practice guidelines. *Osteoporos Int* 1998;**8**(Suppl 4):1–88.

5. Kanis JA, Glüer CC for the Committee of Scientific Advisors, International Osteoporosis Foundation. An update on the diagnosis and assessment of osteoporosis with densitometry. *Osteoporos Int* 2000;**11**:192–202.

6. Kanis JA, Black D, Cooper C et al. A new approach to the development of assessment guidelines for osteoporosis. *Osteoporos Int* 2002;**13**:527–36.

7. World Health Organization. *Assessment of Fracture Risk and its Application to Screening for Postmenopausal Osteoporosis*. Technical Report Series 843. Geneva:WHO, 1994.

8. Kanis JA, Melton LJ, Christiansen C, Johnston CC, Khaltaev N. The diagnosis of osteoporosis. *J Bone Miner Res* 1994;**9**:1137–41.

9. Committee for Proprietary Medicinal Products (CPMP). *Note for Guidance on Involutional Osteoporosis in Women*. London: European Agency for the Evaluation of Medicinal Products, 1997. (CPMP/EWP/552/95)

10. World Health Organization. *Guidelines for Preclinical Evaluation and Clinical Trials in Osteoporosis*. Geneva:WHO, 1998.

11. Liu, Z, Piao J, Pang L, Qing X et al. The diagnostic criteria for primary osteoporosis and the incidence of osteoporosis in China. *J Bone Miner Metab* 2002;**20**:181–9.

12. Kanis JA, Johnell O, Oden A, De Laet C, Mellstrom D. Diagnosis of osteoporosis and fracture threshold in men. *Calcif Tissue Int* 2001;**69**:218–21.

13. De Laet CEDH, Van Hout BA, Burger H, Hofman A, Weel AEAM, Pols HAP. Hip fracture prediction in elderly men and women: validation in the Rotterdam Study. *J Bone Miner Res* 1998;**13**:1587–93.

14. Ross P, Huang C, Davis J et al. Predicting vertebral deformity using bone densitometry at various skeletal sites and calcaneous ultrasound. *Bone* 1995;**16**:325–32.

15. Lunt M, Felsenberg D, Reeve J, Benevolenskaya L, Cannata J, Dequeker J. Bone density variation and its effect

on risk of vertebral deformity in men and women studied in thirteen European Centres: the EVOS Study. *J Bone Miner Res* 1997;**12**: 1883–94.

16. Faulkner KG, von Stetten E, Miller P. Discordance in patient classification using T-scores. *J Clin Densitometry* 1999;**2**:343–50.

17. Arlot ME, Sornay-Rendu E, Garnero P, Vey-Marty B, Delmas PD. Apparent pre- and postmenopausal bone loss evaluated by DXA at different skeletal sites in women: the OFELY cohort. *J Bone Miner Res* 1997;**12**: 683–90.

18. Marshall D, Johnell O, Wedel H. Meta-analysis of how well measures of bone mineral density predict occurrence of osteoporotic fractures. *BMJ* 1996;**312**: 1254–9.

19. Kanis JA, Johnell O, Oden A, De Laet C, Jonsson B, Dawson A. Ten year risk of osteoporotic fracture and the effect of risk factors on screening strategies. *Bone* 2002;**30**:251–8.

20. Kanis JA, Johnell O, Oden A, Jonsson B, De Laet C, Dawson A. Prediction of fracture from low bone mineral density measurements overestimates risk. *Bone* 2000;**26**:387–91.

21. Oden A, Dawson A, Dere W, Johnell O, Jonsson B, Kanis JA. Lifetime risk of hip fracture is underestimated. *Osteoporos Int* 1999;**8**:599–603.

22. Hui SL, Slemenda CW, Johnston CC. Age and bone mass as predictors of fracture in a prospective study. *J Clin Invest* 1988;**81**:1804–9.

23. Kanis JA, Johnell O, Oden A, Dawson A, De Laet C, Jonsson B. Ten year probabilities of osteoporotic fractures according to BMD and diagnostic thresholds. *Osteoporos Int* 2001;**12**: 989–95.

24. Kanis JA. Diagnosis of osteoporosis and assessment of fracture risk. *Lancet* 2002;**359**:1929–36.

25. Kanis JA, McCloskey EV. Evaluation of the risk of hip fracture. *Bone* 1996;**18** (Suppl 3):127–32.

26. Van Staa TP, Leufkens HGM, Abenhaim L, Zhang B, Cooper C. Use of oral corticosteroids and risk of fractures. *J Bone Miner Res* 2001;**15**: 993–1000.

27. Van Staa TP, Leufkens HGM, Cooper C. The epidemiology of cortico-steroid-induced osteoporosis: a meta-analysis. *Osteoporos Int* 2002;**13**: 777–87.

28. Johnell O, De Laet C, Oden A et al. Oral corticosteroids increase fracture risk independently of BMD. *Osteoporos Int* 2001;**13**(Suppl 1):13.

29. Klotzbuecher CM, Ross PD, Landsman PB, Abbot TA, Berger M. Patients with prior fractures have increased risk of future fractures: a summary of the literature and statis-tical synthesis. *J Bone Miner Res* 2000;**15**:721–7.

30. Ross PD, Genant HK, Davis JW, Miller PD, Wasnich RD. Predicting vertebral fracture incidence from prevalent frac-tures and bone density among non black, osteoporotic women. *Osteoporos Int* 1993;**3**:120–6.

31. Delmas PD. The use of biochemical markers of bone turnover in the management of post-menopausal osteoporosis. *Osteoporos Int* 2000;**11** (Suppl 6):S1–S76.

32. Garnero P, Sornay-Rendu E, Claustrat B, Delmas PD. Biochemical markers of bone turnover, endogenous hormones and the risk of fractures in post-menopausal women. The Ofely study. *J Bone Miner Res* 2000;**15**:1526–36.

33. Garnero P, Hauser E, Chapuy MC et al. Markers of bone turnover predict hip fractures in elderly women. The EPIDOS prospective study. *J Bone Min Res* 1996;**11**:1531–8.

34. Hansen M, Overgaard K, Riis B, Christiansen C. Role of peak bone mass and bone loss in post-menopausal osteoporosis: 12 year study. *BMJ* 1991;**303**:961–4.

35. Johnell O, Oden A, De Laet C, Garnero P, Delmas PD, Kanis JA. Biochemical

indices of bone turnover and the assessment of fracture probability. *Osteoporos Int* 2002;**13**:523–6.

36. Dyslipidaemia Advisory Group on behalf of the Scientific Committee of the National Heart Foundation of New Zealand. National Heart Foundation clinical guidelines for the assessment and management of dyslipidaemia. *NZ Med J* 1996;**109**:224–32.

5

The treatment of postmenopausal osteoporosis

Pierre D Delmas

INTRODUCTION

Among various fragility fractures that represent the major complication of osteoporosis, vertebral and hip fractures are associated with significant morbidity and excess mortality. Thus, the prevention and treatment of osteoporosis should be aimed at substantially decreasing the risk of fragility fractures, especially at those sites. In the past 10 years, large double blind placebo controlled trials have been performed in postmenopausal women with osteoporosis, with incident vertebral and nonvertebral fracture as a primary endpoint. These trials have shown that several agents are able to reduce markedly (by 30–50%) the risk of fractures (Table 5.1). This review will focus on such trials whenever available.

Table 5.1 Antifracture efficacy of the most commonly used treatments of postmenopausal osteoporosis in addition to the effects of calcium and/or vitamin D supplementation, as derived from placebo controlled randomized trials

Agents	Vertebral fractures	Nonvertebral fractures
Alendronate	+++	++
Calcitonin (nasal)	+	0
Etidronate	+	0
Fluoride	±	−
Hormone replacement therapy (HRT)	++	++
Ibandronate	+++	0
Menatetrenone (vitamin K2)	+	0
Parathyroid hormone (PTH)	+++	++
Raloxifene	+++	0
Risedronate	+++	++
Strontium ranelate	+++	++
Vitamin D derivatives	±	0

+++, strong evidence; ++, good evidence; +, some evidence; ±, equivocal; 0, no effect; −, negative effects.

Low bone mass is the major risk factor for fractures and the treatment of osteoporosis is focused on agents that will prevent bone loss or even increase bone mass. Osteoporosis, however, is a multi-factorial disease and skeletal fragility results from a variety of factors that are reviewed elsewhere. Thus, optimization of bone health should be implemented throughout life, by age-specific nonpharmacologic intervention that we will review in this chapter.

PHARMACOLOGIC AGENTS

Calcium and vitamin D

Calcium

Calcium is an important nutrient in the prevention and treatment of osteoporosis. Although calcium supplied by dairy products is as effective as calcium supplements, the supplements are necessary in most countries to achieve an adequate calcium intake in osteoporotic patients. Calcium slows the rate of bone loss, particularly in elderly women and in those with a low calcium intake. Some studies have shown some reduction in the incidence of fractures in patients receiving calcium supplements, especially in those with a low dietary calcium intake.[1-3] Calcium is generally prescribed as an adjunct to other drugs for osteoporosis, and in most trials both the active and placebo groups received a calcium supplement, 500–1000 mg/day. Thus, calcium supplementation is useful but not sufficient to treat osteoporotic patients. Calcium supplementation in the order of 500–1500 mg/day is safe. Mild gastrointestinal disturbances, such as constipation, are commonly reported. The risk of kidney stone disease related to increased urinary calcium excretion does not appear to be increased. Bioavailability is greater during meals and varies with different calcium salts, but these factors are probably of little clinical significance.

Vitamin D

In a French study of 3270 institutionalized elderly women (mean age, 84 years) treated for 3 years with calcium (1200 mg/day) and vitamin D (800 IU/day), the probability of hip and all nonvertebral fractures was significantly reduced by 29% and 24%, respectively, as compared to the placebo group.[4,5] Two other smaller studies have shown a trend for a reduction in nonvertebral fractures in elderly men and women treated with annual intramuscular injection of vitamin D or a daily supplement of calcium and vitamin D.[6,7] Conversely, in a Dutch study of 2578 elderly but relatively healthy women with a high calcium intake, a daily supplement with 400 IU of vitamin D given over 3.5 years had no effect on the risk of hip fracture.[8] A recent placebo-controlled study performed in the UK in 2037 men and 649 women aged 65–85 years living in the community showed that 100,000 IU of vitamin D_3 given orally every 4 months over 5 years decreased the risk of clinical fracture (RR 0.78, 95% CI 0.61–0.99), and of the most common osteoporotic sites – hip, wrist, forearm – (RR 0.67, 95% CI 0.48–0.93).[9] Taken together, these data indicate that vitamin D should be used routinely in institutionalized patients because of a high prevalence of vitamin D deficiency (related to low vitamin D intake, low sunshine exposure, and impaired vitamin D synthesis in the skin) but probably also in the elderly living in the community. When compliance is reduced, intramuscular dosing of 150,000–300,000 IU can be administered twice a year. Vitamin D at this dose is safe and does not require monitoring. Conversely, the utility of both calcium and vitamin D supplementation in healthy elderly persons with adequate dairy product intake and normal bone mineral density (BMD) has not been established.

Hormone replacement therapy (HRT)

Several placebo controlled trials have shown that estrogen stops bone loss in early, late and elderly postmenopausal women by inhibiting bone resorption, resulting in 5–10% increase in BMD over a period of 1–3 years.[10–12] There is growing evidence that in elderly women such an increase in BMD can be achieved with smaller doses than those commonly used in early postmenopausal women, in the range of 0.5–1.0 mg of oral 17β-estradiol, 25 μg of transdermal 17β-estradiol, 0.3 mg of conjugated equine estrogens. Calcium supplements may enhance the effect of estrogen on BMD.[13] When HRT is stopped, bone loss probably resumes at the same rate as after the menopause.[14–16]

Several case controlled and cohort studies suggest that HRT decreases the risk of hip fracture by about 30%,[17–19] and two very small placebo controlled studies performed in osteoporotic women suggest a 50% reduction of the risk of spine fractures.[10,20] A recent meta-analysis of 13 randomized placebo controlled trials suggests a 33% reduction in vertebral fracture (95% CI 0.45–0.98).[21] A meta-analysis of 22 randomized trials indicate a 27% reduction in nonvertebral fractures in a pooled analysis (95% CI 0.56–0.94, $p=0.02$), with a 40% reduction for hip and wrist fractures alone.[22] The fact that the reduction in fracture risk appears to be lost within 5 years after HRT withdrawal, regardless of the duration of treatment, raises the issue of the optimal timing and duration of HRT,[23] given the adverse events discussed below. The benefit of HRT on the skeleton has been confirmed in the Women Health Initiative (WHI) performed in 16,608 postmenopausal women aged 50 to 79 years randomized to conjugated equine estrogens (0.625 mg/day) plus medroxyprogesterone acetate (2.5 mg/day) or placebo for 5 years. Although the bone status was unknown at baseline in most of these women, HRT reduced significantly the risk of all clinical fractures (HR 0.76, 95% CI 0.69–0.85) including hip fractures (HR 0.66, 95% CI 0.45–0.98) and clinical vertebral fractures (HR 0.66, 95% CI 0.44–0.98).[24]

HRT has several non-skeletal effects. Women who have undergone hysterectomy can be given estrogen alone. Those with an intact uterus should be given both estrogen and a progestin either in a combined cyclic regimen in women close to menopause, or in a combined continuous regimen, especially in those menopause in for more than five years, to reduce the risk of endometrial carcinoma.[25] With the exception of norethisterone acetate, which has an anabolic effect on bone cells, the addition of a progestin does not influence the effect of estrogen on bone metabolism.[26] Several observational studies have shown a small increase in the risk of breast cancer after 5 to10 years of use,[27,28] confirmed by the WHI study with an HR of 1.26 (95% CI 1.00–1.59).[24] The Million Women Study, a prospective cohort study performed in 1,084,110 women showed in current HRT users an adjusted RR of 1.66 (95% CI 1.58–1.75) for breast cancer and an increased risk of death from breast cancer (RR 1.22, 95% CI 1.00–1.48). Both estrogen only and estrogen plus progestagen significantly increased the risk of breast cancer.[29] Observational studies have suggested a reduction of the risk of coronary heart disease in women taking HRT,[30] but this has not been confirmed in controlled sudies. The HERS study, a secondary prevention trial of coronary heart disease (CHD) in 2321 women, 67 years old, showed no difference between HRT and placebo for the primary outcome (non-fatal myocardial infarction and CHD death) or any of the secondary cardiovascular outcomes during 4 years,[31] a lack of effect which was confirmed after an additional 2.7 years of follow-up.[32] The WHI study showed that the HRT regimen use was associated with a significant increase of CHD (HR 1.29, 95% CI 1.02–1.63) and of stroke (HR 1.41, 95% CI 1.07–1.83).[24] As was shown in the HERS study, the risk of CHD was higher at one year of HRT (HR 1.81, 95% CI 1.09–3.01) and could not be predicted by surrogate markers of cardiovascular disease.[33] HRT increases the risk of deep vein thrombosis and pulmonary embolism.[34] A beneficial effect on cognitive function has been suggested in a retrospective analysis of HRT users but not in randomized controlled studies.[35] In the WHI study, there was no improvement of cognitive function and no benefit of HRT on health-related quality of life.[36]

Selective estrogen receptor modulators (SERMs) and other estrogen analogs

These compounds act as estrogen agonists or antagonists, depending on the target tissue.

Tamoxifen
Tamoxifen, which has long been used for the adjuvant treatment of breast cancer, is an estrogen antagonist in breast tissue but a partial agonist on bone, cholesterol metabolism, and endometrium. Tamoxifen does not entirely prevent bone loss in postmenopausal women[37–39] and increases the risk of endometrial cancer,[40] which precludes its wide use in healthy postmenopausal women.

Raloxifene
Raloxifene is a benzothiophene that competitively inhibits the action of estrogen in the breast and endometrium and acts as an estrogen agonist on

bone and lipid metabolism. In early postmenopausal women, raloxifene prevents postmenopausal bone loss at all skeletal sites, reduces markers of bone turnover to premenopausal level, reduces serum cholesterol concentration and its low density lipoprotein (LDL) fraction, without stimulating the endometrium.[41,42] The MORE study (Multiple Outcomes of Raloxifene Evaluation) performed in 7705 osteoporotic women has shown 30% and 50% reduction of incident vertebral fractures in women with and without prevalent vertebral fractures,[43] respectively, but no effects on nonvertebral fractures (Tables 5.2 and 5.3). There was a 60% reduction in the occurrence of clinical vertebral fracture that was already significant (-62%) after one year of treatment and that was significant both for mild and moderate/severe fractures.[44] In contrast, there was no significant decrease in the rate of nonvertebral fracture with raloxifene at either dose (RR 0.9, 95% CI 0.8–1.1). The results of a 12 month blinded extension of the MORE study was recently published.[45] The 4 year cumulative risks for one or more new vertebral fractures were 0.64 (95% CI 0.53–0.76) with raloxifene 60 mg and 0.57 (97% CI 0.48–0.69) with raloxifene 120 mg/day. In year 4 alone, the reduction of vertebral fracture was significant and not different from the first 3 years. In that study, raloxifene lowered the incidence of breast cancer by 70%.[46,47] The ongoing RUTH study will determine whether the decrease in LDL cholesterol and fibrinogen can result in a reduction in coronary heart disease in high risk populations of postmenopausal women, as shown in a post hoc analysis of the MORE study.[48] Raloxifene does not impair cognitive function in postmenopausal women, with a trend towards less decline in raloxifene-treated women in two tests of vertebral memory and attention as compared to placebo-treated women.[49] Although occurring rarely, thromboembolic disease (venous thrombosis and pulmonary embolism) is significantly increased with raloxifene, with a relative risk similar to that of HRT.[47] Other SERMs are currently under development.

Tibolone

Tibolone is a synthetic steroid that acts on the estrogen, progesterone, and androgen receptor either directly or indirectly through its metabolites, with a different pattern according to the target tissue. Tibolone prevents bone loss in early and late postmenopausal women,[50,51] but its effects on fracture incidence has not been studied. Tibolone reduces menopausal symptoms, appears to be neutral on the endometrium,[52] and does not induce breast tenderness, but the Million Women Study[29] suggests that tibolone increases the risk of breast cancer with an adjusted RR of 1.45 (95% CI 1.25–1.68). Its overall effect on the uterus and the breast should be studied in large and long-term placebo controlled studies. Its effects on cardiovascular disease is unknown.

Bisphosphonates

Bisphosphonates[53] are stable analogs of pyrophosphate characterized by a P-C-P bond. By substituting for hydrogens on the carbon atom, a variety of

Table 5.2 Vertebral fracture (VF) incidence over 3 years (% of patients) and relative risk (RR) with 95% confidence interval (CI) in pivotal trials performed with alendronate, nasal calcitonin, raloxifene, risedronate, and the recombinant 1–34 fragment of human PTH, given at the approved dose in the treatment of postmenopausal osteoporosis.[124,125]

Agent	Trial (ref)	Risk profile	Mean age (years)	No. of patients randomized	Vertebral fracture incidence		
					Placebo (%)	Active agent (%)	RR (95% CI)
Alendronate (5/10 mg)	FIT-1[61]	High (prevalent VF)	71	2027	15	8	0.53 (0.41–0.68)
Calcitonin (200 IU)	PROOF[83]		69	557	15.6	10.8	0.67 (0.47–0.97)
Raloxifene (60 mg)	MORE-2[43]		68	1539	21.2	14.7	0.70 (0.6–0.9)
Risedronate (5 mg)	VERT-US[69]		69	1628	16.3	11.3	0.51 (0.36–0.73)
Risedronate (5 mg)	VERT-MN[70]		71	815	29	18.1	0.59 (0.43–0.82)
rhPTH(1–34) (20 µg)	Neer et al.[85]		69	892	14*	5*	0.35 (0.22–0.55)*
Alendronate (5/10 mg)	FIT-2[62]	Low (without prevalent VF)	68	4432 / 1631**	2.7 / 4.2**	1.5 / 2.1**	0.56 (0.39–0.8) / 0.50 (0.31–0.82)**
Raloxifene (60 mg)	MORE-1[43]		65	3012	4.5	2.3	0.50 (0.4–0.8)

The 3 year incidence was extrapolated from 4.2 years in FIT-2, and 5 years in PROOF. Results obtained with ibandronate and strontium ranelate have been published in abstract form and full data are not yet available.

*incidence and RR at 21 months. **in the subgroup of women with a T-score ≤ -2.5

Table 5.3 Hip fracture incidence over 3 years (% of patients) and relative risk (RR) with 95% confidence interval (CI) in pivotal trials performed with alendronate, nasal calcitonin, PTH, raloxifene and risedronate in the treatment of postmenopausal osteoporosis.[124,125]

Agent	Trial (ref)	Risk profile	Mean age (years)	No. of patients randomized	Placebo (%)	Active agent (%)	RR (95% CI)
						Hip fracture incidence	
Risedronate (2.5 and 5 mg)	HIP[60]	70–80 years old with osteoporosis	74	5445	3.2 5.7*	1.9 2.3*	0.6 (0.4–0.9) 0.4 (0.2–0.8)
		>80 years old with/without osteoporosis	83	3886	5.1	4.2	0.8 (0.6–1.2)
Alendronate (5/10 mg)	FIT-1[61]	Patients with vertebral fractures	71	2027	2.2	1.1	0.49 (0.23–0.99)
Calcitonin (200 IU)	PROOF[83]		69	557	1.8	1.2	0.5 (0.2–1.6)
Risedronate (5 mg)	VERT-US[69]		69	1628	1.8	1.4	n.a.
Risedronate (5 mg)	VERT-MN[70]		71	815	2.7	2.2	n.a.
rhPTH(1–34) (20 µg)	Neer et al.[85]		69	892	0.74**	0.037**	n.a.
Raloxifene (60 and 120 mg)	MORE[43]	Osteoporosis (T-score ≤ −2.5) with/without vertebral fractures	67	7705	0.7	0.8	1.1 (0.6–1.9)
Alendronate (5/10 mg)	FIT-2[62]	T-score ≤ −2.5 T-score ≤ −1.6	n.a. 68	1631 4432	1.6 0.8	0.72 0.65	0.44 (0.18–0.97) 0.79 (0.43–1.44)

The 3 year incidence was extrapolated from 4.2 years in FIT-2, and 5 years in PROOF. Results obtained with ibandronate and strontium ranelate have been published in abstract form and full data are not yet available.
*in the subgroup with prevalent vertebral fractures. **incidence at 21 months; n.a., not available.

bisphosphonates have been synthesized, the potency of which depends on the length and structure of the side chain. Bisphosphonates have a strong affinity for bone apatite, which is the basis for their clinical use. Bisphosphonates are potent inhibitors of bone resorption, reducing the recruitment and activity of osteoclasts and increasing their apoptosis, through a molecular mechanism recently identified. The oral bioavailability of bisphosphonates is low, between 1% and 3% of the dose ingested, and is impaired by food, calcium, iron, coffee, tea and orange juice. They are quickly cleared from plasma, with approximately 50% deposited in bone and 50% excreted in urine. The half-life of bisphosphonates in bone is very long, several years in the human skeleton, but varies significantly from compound to compound. The safety profile of bisphosphonates is favorable. Minor to moderate gastrointestinal discomfort has been reported for all bisphosphonates (dyspepsia, abdominal pain, diarrhea), rarely leading to discontinuation. Rare cases of esophagitis have been reported with alendronate.[54] Etidronate, but not other bisphosphonates, can induce a mineralization defect of bone after prolonged use, especially in patients with renal insufficiency. Their effects on fractures are summarized in Tables 5.2 and 5.3.

Etidronate
Etidronate was the first bisphosphonate to be developed. Given in an intermittent regimen (400 mg/day, 15 days every 3 months), etidronate increases spine BMD by about 4%, with a reduction of vertebral fracture rate at two years,[55,56] that was no longer significant after 3 years of treatment in one of the two studies.[57] A meta-analysis of controlled etidronate trials performed over 1–4 years suggested a reduction of vertebral fractures with a relative risk of 0.63 (95% CI 0.44–0.92) but no effect on nonvertebral fractures.[58]

Alendronate
Alendronate prevents postmenopausal bone loss.[59,60] A study (FIT-1) in 2025 osteoporotic women with at least one prevalent vertebral fracture treated with alendronate 5 mg daily for two years followed by 10 mg daily during a third year demonstrated a significant 50% reduction of vertebral, wrist and hip fractures compared to the placebo.[61] Women with a low BMD but without vertebral fracture at baseline (FIT-2) were treated with alendronate for four years with the same placebo controlled design. There was a small decrease of clinical fracture incidence with alendronate that did not reach significance ($p=0.07$), while the incidence of new vertebral fractures was significantly reduced by the treatment.[62] When the analysis was restricted to those patients having osteoporosis according to the WHO criteria, that is with a BMD below 2.5 standard deviations below the mean value of healthy premenopausal women (T-score ≤-2.5), the reduction of all types of clinical fractures was significant, but there was no effect in those with higher BMD.[62] A pooled analysis of osteoporotic women from both FIT studies shows that the reduction of the risk of fracture under alendronate occurs early, within 12–18 months.[63] Another placebo controlled study in 1908 postmenopausal women with a low BMD

(T-score ≤-2) showed a 47% reduction in the risk of nonvertebral fracture after one year of alendronate 10 mg/day.[64] The optimal duration of treatment is unknown. A recent study suggests that seven years of alendronate is safe, but there may not be additional benefit after five years, based on changes of BMD and bone turnover markers.[65] Alendronate given once a week at the dose of 70 mg has the same efficacy as 10 mg daily to increase BMD and reduce bone turnover, with a good safety profile,[66,67] and may improve the long term compliance, a challenge in such a chronic disease.

Risedronate

Risedronate prevents postmenopausal bone loss.[68] Risedronate 5 mg/day reduced significantly the cumulative incidence of patients with new vertebral fractures by 41% over three years and by 65% after the first year in 2400 women with prevalent vertebral fractures.[69] In another study including 1226 patients with severe osteoporosis (at least two prevalent vertebral fractures) risedronate resulted in a 49% reduction of vertebral fracture incidence at 3 years[70] and the effect was maintained in a 2 year placebo-controlled extension performed in a subgroup of these patients.[71] The analysis of pooled data from both studies showed a 90% reduction of the risk of multiple vertebral fractures.[72] A post hoc analysis in 640 patients with osteoporosis (i.e. a T-score ≤-2.5) but without prevalent vertebral fracture taken from various placebo controlled trials showed that risedronate 5 mg/day reduces the risk of the first vertebral fracture by 75% ($p=0.002$).[73] The overall incidence of nonvertebral fracture in both studies was reduced by 30–40%.[69,70] The effects of risedronate on hip fracture has been assessed in 5445 women aged 70–79 years with osteoporosis defined by a low BMD and in 3896 women over 80 years of age that were mainly recruited on the basis of clinical risk factors for falls, without BMD assessment in most of them.[74] The overall analysis showed a 30% reduction of hip fracture ($p=0.02$) with risedronate over three years. In the first group, the reduction of hip fractures was larger (40%), reaching 60% in those with prevalent vertebral fractures. In contrast, there was no significant reduction in the second group, stressing the need to target bisphosphonates to those women that have osteoporosis as confirmed by BMD measurement. Risedronate 35 mg once a week is equivalent to 5 mg daily.

Other bisphosphonates

Clodronate was developed more than 20 years ago and is still widely used for the treatment of malignant bone diseases. In a study of 677 patients with osteoporosis, including postmenopausal, secondary, and male osteoporosis, clodronate 800 mg/day decreased significantly the incidence of new vertebral fractures by 46%.[75] **Tiludronate** is a bisphosphonate used in several countries for the treatment of Paget's disease of bone. However, its development for osteoporosis has been discontinued because of the lack of evidence of fracture reduction in large phase III trials at the dose that was tested. Oral daily **pamidronate** may be efficient in osteoporosis but is associated with a high incidence of upper gastrointestinal adverse events.[76] Intravenous infusion of pamidronate, commonly used in malignant bone disease and in Paget's disease of bone, has been shown to increase BMD at the spine and hip when infused in osteoporotic patients every three months.[77] No fracture data are available. **Ibandronate** and **zoledronate**, two new potent bisphosphonates, are currently under investigation in phase III trials. A single intravenous injection of 4 mg of zoledronate has been shown to increase spine BMD by 4% and to decrease bone resorption markers by 60% one year after the injection, suggesting a long lasting supression of bone turnover.[78] In postmenopausal osteoporotic patients, oral ibandronate given either daily 2.5 mg or intermittently – with a drug-free interval of 2 months and with a cumulative dose similar to the daily regimen – induced a 50–60% reduction of the risk of new vertebral fractures without a significant reduction of nonvertebral fractures.[79] Other intermittent regimens are currently being tested.

Calcitonin

Calcitonin, a peptide produced by thyroid C cells, reduces bone resorption by directly inhibiting the osteoclast activity. When given by subcutaneous or intramuscular injection, the tolerance is sometimes poor (nausea, facial flushes, diarrhea), while the tolerance of the intranasal route of salmon calcitonin is excellent. The minimum intranasal dose to have a significant effect on BMD is 200 IU/day. Calcitonin is less effective in preventing cortical bone loss than cancellous bone loss in postmenopausal women.[80,81] A small controlled study in osteoporotic women suggested a reduction in new fractures.[82] In the PROOF (Prevent Recurrence Of Osteoporotic Fractures) study, which is a five year double blind randomized placebo controlled study of 1255 postmenopausal women with osteoporosis, 200 IU/day of intranasal salmon calcitonin appeared to significantly reduce the rate of vertebral, but not peripheral, fractures by about 30% in comparison to the placebo, but 60% of subjects were lost to follow up, doses of 100 IU and 400 IU had no effect, and no consistent effect on BMD and bone turnover markers were seen.[83]

Parathyroid hormone (PTH)

The excess of PTH secretion as well as continuous intravenous infusion result in increased bone resorption and bone loss. In contrast, there is compelling evidence in a range of species made osteoporotic by gonadectomy that intermittent PTH injection restores bone strength by stimulating new bone formation at the periosteal (outer) and endosteal (inner) bone surfaces, thickening the cortices and existing trabeculae, and perhaps increasing trabecular numbers and their connectivity.[84] In a recent double blind placebo controlled prospective study in 1637 postmenopausal women with prior vertebral fractures, daily treatment with either 20 μg or 40 μg of subcutaneous recombinant human PTH(1–34) for a median of 19 months markedly reduced the incidence of new vertebral fractures, with a relative risk of 0.35 and 0.31 for these respective doses.[85] The incidence of nonvertebral fragility fractures was reduced by 53% with either dose (Tables 5.2 and 5.3). The increase in BMD with the 20 μg and 40 μg doses were 9% and 12% at the spine, 3% and 6% at the femoral neck, and 2% and 4% at the total body after 21 months of observation. The highest dose occasionally caused nausea and headache. There was a dose dependent increase in serum calcium within the first 4–6 hours after injection, that was mild and transient, occurring in 11% of patients with the 20 μg dose. In long-term toxicologic studies, high doses of PTH induce osteosarcomas in rats but not in monkeys. In clinical studies involving about 1000 patients, treatment with PTH or its fragments for up to three years has not increased the incidence of tumors in bone or other tissues. PTH, 20 μg/day for 18 months, has been registered in the USA and in Europe.

Other treatments

Vitamin D analogs. Alfacalcidol and calcitriol are used in some countries for the treatment of osteoporosis. Both induce a small increase in BMD that appears to be limited to the spine, and data on the reduction of fracture risk are scarce and conflicting.[86–89] In a large randomized study that was not placebo controlled,[90] the rate of vertebral fracture was reduced in osteoporotic patients receiving calcitriol in comparison to those receiving calcium alone because of an unusual increase of the annual fracture rate in the calcium group with time. No study has compared the effect of vitamin D derivatives versus calcium plus vitamin D on fracture risk. Vitamin D derivatives expose patients to hypercalcemia and hypercalciuria. Serum and urine calcium levels should be monitored, and the dose adapted.

Fluoride salt. Fluoride is incorporated into the hydroxyapatite component of bone. It stimulates osteoblast recruitment and activity, thus increasing the rate of bone formation. In humans, sodium fluoride increases spine BMD linearly with time, with little effect at the hip. Two large placebo controlled trials[91,92] of fluoride with vertebral fracture incidence as a primary endpoint, using different preparations and dose of fluoride salts, have shown that fluoride does not decrease vertebral fracture rate, in contrast to an earlier report.[93] There is some evidence that it may have an adverse effect on the risk of hip fracture. The use of fluoride in the treatment of postmenopausal osteoporosis cannot be recommended.

Vitamin K. Serum concentrations of circulating vitamin K, especially of the K_2 moieties, decrease with ageing and is lower in patients with hip fractures. In the nurses health study cohort, low intakes of vitamin K has been associated with an increased risk of hip fracture. The consequences of this deficiency on bone metabolism are still speculative, but probably explain the increase in the under-carboxylated fraction of serum osteocalcin, a marker of bone fragility in the elderly.[94] Treatment of osteoporotic patients with menatetrenone, a vitamin

K$_2$ compound, has been associated with improved BMD[95] and is approved for the treatment of osteoporosis in Japan. A positive effect on fragility fractures is suggested by a small controlled study.[96]

Strontium ranelate. Strontium ranelate is a new antiosteoporotic agent which has recently received its approval in the European Union for the treatment of postmenopausal osteoporosis to reduce the risk of vertebral and hip fractures. Strontium ranelate is the first antiosteoporotic agent that appears to simultaneously increase bone formation and decrease bone resorption.[97,98] Results from a phase III clinical trial, carried out in 1649 postmenopausal women show that strontium ranelate significantly reduces the risk of new vertebral fractures by 49% after one year and 41% over 3 years.[98] Clinical vertebral fracture risk was also reduced by 52% in the first year and in the long term. Results from a second large scale phase-III clinical trial have shown that strontium ranelate reduces the risk of nonvertebral fractures in postmenopausal women, as well as the risk of hip fracture in a subgroup with low BMD.[99] In both these trials BMD was significantly increased at the lumbar spine, femoral neck and total hip. Strontium ranelate was well tolerated, particularly at an upper-gastrointestinal level.[98] The results of these trials show that strontium ranelate should be useful in the treatment of postmenopausal osteoporosis.

Growth hormone. Growth hormone has been used for its alleged bone and muscle anabolic properties, but it has produced conflicting results in the prevention of bone loss in postmenopausal osteoporosis.

Thiazide diuretics. Thiazide diuretics reduce tubular reabsorption of calcium and may decrease bone turnover and bone loss but their role in the management of osteoporosis has not been established.

Ipriflavone. Ipriflavone is a synthetic compound that belongs to the family of isoflavones. Although preliminary results suggested that it could prevent bone loss, it does not appear to reduce the incidence of fractures in osteoporotic women.[100]

Statins. Statins increase bone mass and strength in rats,[101] but epidemiologic studies relating their use to the occurrence of fractures are inconclusive.

NONPHARMACOLOGIC INTERVENTION

Nutrition

Good nutrition and a balanced diet with adequate calories are important for normal growth. Calcium is the most important nutrient for attaining adequate peak bone mass, but there is no universal consensus on the daily calcium requirement by age. The 1994 Consensus Development Conference on

Optimal Calcium Intake recommended 1200–1500 mg/day for adolescents, 1000 mg/day for adults up to 65 years of age, 1500 mg/day for postmenopausal women not receiving estrogen and in the elderly.[102] A recent NIH panel has reinforced the importance of adequate calcium intake.[103] Although most studies have shown a beneficial effect of calcium supplement as discussed above, the long-term effect of a high dietary calcium intake on bone health is unclear. Conversely, there seems to be a threshold of calcium intake, around 400 mg/day, under which increasing calcium intake appears to be beneficial and necessary, both in children and in women older than 60 years.

Vitamin D is essential for the intestinal absorption of calcium and, as discussed above, the serum levels of 25-hydroxyvitamin D decline with ageing. Several studies suggest that the daily intake of vitamin D should be around 400–800 IU/day if sunlight exposure is low. An adequate protein intake is critical in the frail elderly.

Exercise

There is evidence that physical activity early in life contributes to higher peak bone mass.[104] Various exercises, including walking, weight training and high impact exercises, induce a small (1–2%) increase in BMD at some but not all skeletal sites, which is not sustained once the exercise program is stopped. Both clinical trials and observational studies suggest that load bearing exercise is more effective on bone mass than other types of exercise.[104] Fitness might indirectly preserve individuals from fractures by improving mobility and muscle function and reducing the risk of falls.[105] Observational studies suggest that regular exercise and recreational activity decrease hip and lower extremity fracture risk but increases the risk of wrist fracture. After a vertebral fracture, a supervised exercise program to maintain strength and flexibility of the thoracic and lumbar spine is recommended in the elderly. It is also critical to develop specific interventions aimed at preventing falls and their consequences in this group.[106] Controlled studies have shown that exercise can increase muscle mass and strength, and reduce the risk of falls by approximately 25% in frail elderly.[107] So far, no controlled study has shown that such exercise programs can reduce the risk of fracture regardless of age.

Orthopedic management of osteoporotic fractures

The early surgical management of hip fractures is essential to decrease the mortality rate, and to improve perioperative morbidity, which is quite significant especially in the frail elderly. The surgical treatment of peripheral fragility fractures does not require specific procedures as fracture healing in osteoporotic patients is normal for their age. In patients with major pain related to a crushed vertebra, vertebral plasty using injection of polymetalmetacrylate cement into the vertebral body has been suggested.[108] It may have a beneficial effect on acute pain, but the long-term effect of such a procedure on the subsequent risk of fractures of adjacent vertebrae needs to be assessed in a controlled study.

Other measures

Drugs predisposing to osteoporosis, such as chronic corticosteroid therapy, should be avoided as much as possible. In addition to an exercise program, a strategy to decrease the risk of falls in the frail elderly should be implemented. Visual impairment and cataract should be detected and treated, as visual impairment increase the risk of falls. Whenever possible, the use of drugs that increase the risk of falling should be reduced, such as basodiazepine, hypnotics, antidepressant agents, and medications that can induce hypotension. Patients should be instructed to avoid slippery floors and inadequate lights at home. Finally, two control studies performed in the institutionalized elderly have shown that the risk of hip fracture could be reduced by as much as 50% with the use of energy-absorbing external hip protectors,[109,110] but the long-term compliance with these devices is unknown.

WHICH AGENT FOR WHICH PATIENT?

The decision-making process concerning treatment of postmenopausal osteoporosis should be based on the assessment of the patient's risk of fracture and on the efficacy and tolerance of the drugs likely to be prescribed. As reviewed elsewhere, fracture risk depends mainly on the magnitude of bone loss assessed by the level of BMD at the spine and hip, on age, on the presence or not of previous fragility fractures, especially of the spine, and to a lesser extent, on some other clinical risk factors that might be influenced by bone-specific agents. Based on several epidemiologic studies, algorithms are currently being derived that will establish the 10 year probability of all low trauma fractures (including spine, hip, and other sites) according to age, history of fractures, the level of bone mass assessed by dual-energy X-ray absorptiometry or other relevant techniques and to the level of bone resorption assessed by specific biochemical markers. Those algorithms that provide an absolute risk of fractures should be useful for the clinician to make a treatment decision. In general, those with higher absolute risk will derive greater benefit. However, bisphosphonate trials suggest that a reduction of nonvertebral fracture is only advised in those patients with osteoporosis based on BMD level, regardless of the absolute fracture risk due to other risk factors. In addition to an adequate intake of calcium and vitamin D, pharmacological options for the prevention and/or treatment of osteoporosis include bisphosphonates (alendronate, risedronate), raloxifene, HRT, calcitonin, and in some countries PTH. The decision on when and how to treat depends on the clinical presentation as discussed below.

Patients with fractures

Vertebral fracture is probably the most common fragility fracture in post-menopausal women in their 60s and 70s. Other etiologies, such as malignancy, need to be ruled out by adequate clinical and biological investigation. Although BMD measurement is not necessary for treatment decision, it is usually performed, confirming the existence of a low BMD. These patients require treatment, as there is good evidence that the risk of further vertebral fractures is extremely high, around 20% in the 12 months following a recent vertebral fracture.[111] Alendronate, risedronate, raloxifene and PTH are the best treatment options, based on the scientific evidence. Because of its high cost and constraint of administration, PTH is likely to be mostly used in patients with multiple vertebral fractures (i.e. in those at highest risk).

In patients with other **low trauma fractures**, the existence of skeletal fragility underlying the fracture needs to be documented by a BMD measurement. In case of a low BMD (T-score ≤ -1) treatment should be considered, based on the type of fracture (all hip fractures should be treated, while fractures of the toes and fingers are usually nonosteoporotic), on age, additional risk factors and current BMD, as fracture risk doubles for every decrease of BMD of one standard deviation.

Women without a history of low trauma fractures

If a postmenopausal woman has osteoporosis according to the WHO definition (i.e. T-score ≤ -2.5 at the spine and/or hip), the risk of fracture is high enough to justify a treatment (alendronate, raloxifene or risedronate). In the case of osteopenia (T-scores between -1 and -2.5) prevention of osteoporosis might be considered if BMD is in the lower range (i.e. < -2) or if there are other clinical risk factors for fractures.

The choice of treatment is influenced by age. Thus, HRT is the treatment of choice to prevent bone loss in early postmenopausal women with menopausal symptoms but at the lowest dose effective to reduce hot flushes and for a duration as short as possible, given its effects on the breast and cardiovascular disease. Raloxifene is an attractive alternative for reducing the risk of vertebral fractures in middle and late postmenopausal women, especially if concerned about the risk of breast cancer. Bisphosphonates have no extra skeletal benefits, but have the ability to reduce the risk of vertebral, hip, and other types of fractures. Thus, although they can be used at any age in postmenopausal women, they appear to be the first choice in women at highest risk of nonvertebral fracture including elderly women, when the risk of hip fracture is increasing exponentially with age.

How to monitor treatment?

As for most chronic diseases, the long-term compliance to osteoporosis therapy appears to be poor. Thus, the goal of monitoring should be to increase adherence to the treatment regimen, as well as to determine the response to treatment. Because fracture events are uncommon, they cannot be used for such monitoring. BMD measurement, especially at the spine, is commonly repeated at a two year interval, but the relatively low signal-to-noise ratio of this technique with anti-resorptive therapies does not allow easy detection of responders and non-responders to therapy. If a non-response (i.e. a significant decrease of BMD is detected), it should be confirmed by a subsequent measurement, in order to minimize the statistical phenomenon of regression to the mean.[112] The use of biochemical markers of formation and resorption has been proposed as a monitoring tool with anti-resorptive therapies. Several studies have shown a significant inverse correlation between the short-term (3–6 months) decrease in bone turnover markers and the 2–3 year increase in BMD at various skeletal sites with HRT and bisphosphonate therapy.[113–115] Cut-off for these decreases for a given marker and treatment that will identify responders and non-responders with adequate sensitivity and specificity have been proposed recently by the Committee of Scientific Advisors of the International Osteoporosis Foundation.[116] Studies are currently underway to correlate short-term changes in bone turnover markers with the probability of future fractures in women with osteoporosis, and such an association has already been reported for raloxifene[117] and risedronate.[118] Whether BMD measurement and/or bone markers are used for monitoring treatment response, it remains to be demonstrated that such an approach improves the long-term compliance to treatment.

PERSPECTIVES AND CONCLUSIONS

Although there are now several therapies that have been shown to reduce substantially the risk of fragility fractures, the mechanisms underlying this effect are still poorly understood. Most anti-resorptive therapies induce a 2–10% increase in spinal BMD and the reduction of the risk of fracture is greater than expected from that change of BMD.[119] In addition, raloxifene increases spinal BMD by only 2–3%,[41] as compared to 8% with alendronate,[120] despite modest differences in vertebral fracture rate. The increase in BMD appears to be mainly related to an increase in the amount of mineral per unit of bone, as shown by quantitative microradiography, rather than to an increase in true bone mass.[121] Decreased bone turnover is another determinant of fracture reduction, as shown by clinical studies, and there are probably other mechanisms that are important, involving changes in bone structure and biology that may vary according to the skeletal envelope.[122] Our incomplete understanding of the mechanism by which anti-resorptive agents improve skeletal strengths at some – but not necessarily at all – skeletal sites deserve further investigation.

Because PTH acts by mechanisms that are totally different from anti-resorptive therapy, it also opens new perspectives of combination therapy for patients with severe osteoporosis. Anti-resorptive agents appear to maintain bone mass, structure and strength when PTH is stopped in animal models, and drugs like bisphosphonate, raloxifene or HRT may be useful to maintain the effects of PTH when it is withdrawn. Concomitant therapy with estrogen does not appear to blunt the anabolic effects of PTH in postmenopausal women,[123] but there is no evidence that this combination produces a higher bone mass or greater bone strength than PTH alone. Combination of bisphosphonates (alendronate or risedronate) with HRT or raloxifene has been shown to induce an increase in BMD slightly higher than either treatment alone, but there is no evidence that it results in a more efficient prevention of fracture.

Until today, only a small proportion of patients with a fragility fracture are treated despite efficient treatments, because of the low awareness of its consequences. Because fractures are associated with increased morbidity and mortality, treatment should be offered to postmenopausal women at high risk of fragility fractures, that is:

(i)   Women with vertebral fractures
(ii)   Those with nonvertebral fractures associated with low BMD
(iii) Those with osteoporosis as defined by the WHO, i.e. a T-score ≤ -2.5.

The most rigorously investigated drugs reported to reduce spine fractures are alendronate, raloxifene, risedronate and rhPTH. The most rigorously investigated drugs reported to reduce nonvertebral fractures, of which the hip is the major concern, are vitamin D with or without calcium in institutionalized elderly, alendronate, risedronate and rhPTH in the community. Because of its marked reduction of vertebral and nonvertebral fractures, PTH will be an interesting alternative in patients with severe osteoporosis, when available.

Prevention of osteoporosis should be decided on a case basis, according to age, the level of BMD and some additional risk factors. Short-term HRT is an alternative in early postmenopausal women with menopausal symptoms, while asymptomatic women should benefit from raloxifene, or a bisphosphonate for those with a high risk of nonvertebral fractures.

REFERENCES

1. Dawson-Hughes B, Dallal GE, Krall EA et al. A controlled trial of the effect of calcium supplementation on bone density in postmenopausal women. *N Engl J Med* 1990;**323**: 878–83.
2. Reid IR, Ames RW, Evans MC et al. Long-term effects of calcium supplementation on bone loss and fractures in postmenopausal women: a randomized controlled trial. *Am J Med* 1995; **98**:331–5.
3. Recker RR, Hinders S, Davies KM et al. Correcting calcium nutritional deficiency prevents spine fractures in elderly women. *J Bone Miner Res* 1996; **11**:1961–6.
4. Chapuy MC, Arlot ME, Duboeuf F et al. Vitamin D3 and calcium to prevent hip fractures in the elderly women. *N Engl J Med* 1992;**327**:1637–42.
5. Chapuy MC, Arlot ME, Delmas PD, Meunier PJ. Effect of calcium and cholecalciferol treatment for three years on hip fractures in elderly women. *BMJ* 1994;**308**:1081–2.
6. Heikinheimo RJ, Inkovaara JA, Harju EJ et al. Annual injection of vitamin D and fractures of aged bones. *Calcif Tissue Int* 1992;**51**:105–10.
7. Dawson-Hughes B, Harris SS, Krall EA, Dallal GE. Effect of calcium and vitamin D supplementation on bone density in men and women 65 years of age or older. *N Engl J Med* 1997;**337**: 670–6.
8. Lips P, Graafmans WC, Ooms ME et al. Vitamin D supplementation and fracture incidence in elderly persons. A randomized, placebo-controlled clinical trial. *Ann Intern Med* 1996; **124**:400–6.
9. Trivedi DP, Doll R, Khaw KT. Effect of four monthly oral vitamin D3 (cholecalciferol) supplementation on fractures and mortality in men and women living in the community: randomised double blind controlled trial. *BMJ* 2003;**326**:469.
10. Lindsay R, Hart DM, Forrest C, Baird C. Prevention of spinal osteoporosis in oophorectomised women. *Lancet* 1980;**2**:1151–4.
11. The Writing Group for the PEPI. Effects of hormone therapy on bone mineral density: results from the postmenopausal estrogen/progestin interventions (PEPI) trial. *JAMA* 1996;**276**: 1389–96.
12. Pors Nielsen S, Barenholdt O, Hermansen F, Munk-Jensen N. Magnitude and pattern of skeletal response to long term continuous and cyclic sequential oestrogen/progestin treatment. *Br J Obstet Gynaecol* 1994; **101**:319–24.
13. Nieves JW, Komar L, Cosman F, Lindsay R. Calcium potentiates the effect of estrogen and calcitonin on bone mass: review and analysis. *Am J Clin Nutr* 1998;**67**:18–24.
14. Christiansen C, Christensen MS, Transbol I. Bone mass in postmenopausal women after withdrawal of oestrogen/gestagen replacement therapy. *Lancet* 1981;**1**:459–61.
15. Felson DT, Zhang Y, Hannan MT et al. The effect of postmenopausal estrogen therapy on bone density in elderly women. *N Engl J Med* 1993;**329**: 1141–6.
16. Lindsay R, Hart DM, Fogelman I. Bone mass after withdrawal of oestrogen replacement. *Lancet* 1981;**1**:729.
17. Kiel DP, Felson DT, Anderson JJ et al. Hip fracture and the use of estrogens in postmenopausal women. The Framingham Study. *N Engl J Med* 1987;**317**:1169–74.
18. Maxim P, Ettinger B, Spitalny GM. Fracture protection provided by long-term estrogen treatment. *Osteoporos Int* 1995;**5**:23–29.
19. Paganini-Hill A, Ross RK, Gerkins VR et al. Menopausal estrogen therapy and hip fractures. *Ann Intern Med* 1981;**95**:28–31.
20. Lufkin EG, Wahner HW, O'Fallon WM et al. Treatment of postmenopausal osteoporosis with transdermal estrogen. *Ann Intern Med* 1992; **117**:1–9.

21. Torgerson DJ, Bell-Syer SE. Hormone replacement therapy and prevention of vertebral fractures: a meta-analysis of randomised trials. *BMC Musculoskelet Disord* 2001;**2**:7.

22. Torgerson DJ, Bell-Syer SE. Hormone replacement therapy and prevention of nonvertebral fractures: a meta-analysis of randomized trials. *JAMA* 2001;**285**:2891–7.

23. Cauley JA, Seeley DG, Ensrud K et al. Estrogen replacement therapy and fractures in older women. Study of Osteoporotic Fractures Research Group. *Ann Intern Med* 1995;**122**: 9–16.

24. Rossouw JE, Anderson GL, Prentice RL et al. Risks and benefits of estrogen plus progestin in healthy postmenopausal women: principal results from the Women's Health Initiative randomized controlled trial. *JAMA* 2002;**288**:321–33.

25. Beresford SA, Weiss NS, Voigt LF, McKnight B. Risk of endometrial cancer in relation to use of oestrogen combined with cyclic progestagen therapy in postmenopausal women. *Lancet* 1997;**349**:458–61.

26. Delmas PD. Hormone replacement therapy in the prevention and treatment of osteoporosis. *Osteoporos Int* 1997;**7**(Suppl 1):S3–S7.

27. Bergkvist L, Persson I. Hormone replacement therapy and breast cancer. A review of current knowledge. *Drug Saf* 1996;**15**:360–70.

28. Colditz GA, Hankinson SE, Hunter DJ et al. The use of estrogens and progestins and the risk of breast cancer in postmenopausal women. *N Engl J Med* 1995;**332**:1589–93.

29. Beral V. Breast cancer and hormone-replacement therapy in the Million Women Study. *Lancet* 2003;**362**: 419–27.

30. Grodstein F, Stampfer MJ, Manson JE et al. Postmenopausal estrogen and progestin use and the risk of cardiovascular disease. *N Engl J Med* 1996; **335**:453–61.

31. Hulley S, Grady D, Bush T et al. Randomized trial of estrogen plus progestin for secondary prevention of coronary heart disease in postmenopausal women. Heart and Estrogen/progestin Replacement Study (HERS) Research Group. *JAMA* 1998;**280**:605–13.

32. Grady D, Herrington D, Bittner V et al. Cardiovascular disease outcomes during 6.8 years of hormone therapy: Heart and Estrogen/progestin Replacement Study follow-up (HERS II). *JAMA* 2002;**288**:49–57.

33. Manson JE, Hsia J, Johnson KC et al. Estrogen plus progestin and the risk of coronary heart disease. *N Engl J Med* 2003;**349**:523–34.

34. Grodstein F, Stampfer MJ, Goldhaber SZ et al. Prospective study of exogenous hormones and risk of pulmonary embolism in women. *Lancet* 1996; **348**:983–7.

35. Tang MX, Jacobs D, Stern Y et al. Effect of oestrogen during menopause on risk and age at onset of Alzheimer's disease. *Lancet* 1996;**348**:429–32.

36. Hays J, Ockene JK, Brunner RL et al. Effects of estrogen plus progestin on health-related quality of life. *N Engl J Med* 2003;**348**:1839–54.

37. Love RR, Mazess RB, Barden HS et al. Effects of tamoxifen on bone mineral density in postmenopausal women with breast cancer. *N Engl J Med* 1992; **326**:852–6.

38. Grey AB, Stapleton JP, Evans MC et al. The effect of the antiestrogen tamoxifen on bone mineral density in normal late postmenopausal women. *Am J Med* 1995;**99**:636–41.

39. Delmas PD, Balena R, Confravreux E et al. Bisphosphonate risedronate prevents bone loss in women with artificial menopause due to chemotherapy of breast cancer: a double-blind, placebo-controlled study. *J Clin Oncol* 1997;**15**:955–62.

40. Fisher B, Costantino JP, Redmond CK et al. Endometrial cancer in tamoxifen-treated breast cancer patients: findings from the National Surgical Adjuvant Breast and Bowel Project (NSABP) B-14. *J Natl Cancer Inst* 1994;**86**:527–37.

41. Delmas PD, Bjarnason NH, Mitlak BH

et al. Effects of raloxifene on bone mineral density, serum cholesterol concentrations, and uterine endometrium in postmenopausal women. *N Engl J Med* 1997;**337**:1641–7.

42. Walsh BW, Kuller LH, Wild RA et al. Effects of raloxifene on serum lipids and coagulation factors in healthy postmenopausal women. *JAMA* 1998; **279**:1445–51.

43. Ettinger B, Black DM, Mitlak BH et al. Reduction of vertebral fracture risk in postmenopausal women with osteoporosis treated with raloxifene: results from a 3-year randomized clinical trial. Multiple Outcomes of Raloxifene Evaluation (MORE) Investigators. *JAMA* 1999;**282**:637–45.

44. Siris E, Adachi JD, Lu Y et al. Effects of raloxifene on fracture severity in postmenopausal women with osteoporosis: results from the MORE study. Multiple Outcomes of Raloxifene Evaluation. *Osteoporos Int* 2002;**13**: 907–13.

45. Delmas PD, Ensrud KE, Adachi JD et al. Efficacy of raloxifene on vertebral fracture risk reduction in postmenopausal women with osteoporosis: four-year results from a randomized clinical trial. *J Clin Endocrinol Metab* 2002;**87**:3609–17.

46. Cummings SR, Eckert S, Krueger KA et al. The effect of raloxifene on risk of breast cancer in postmenopausal women: results from the MORE randomized trial. Multiple Outcomes of Raloxifene Evaluation. *JAMA* 1999;**281**:2189–97.

47. Cauley JA, Norton L, Lippman ME et al. Continued breast cancer risk reduction in postmenopausal women treated with raloxifene: 4-year results from the MORE trial. Multiple outcomes of raloxifene evaluation. *Breast Cancer Res Treat* 2001;**65**: 125–34.

48. Barrett-Connor E, Grady D, Sashegyi A et al. Raloxifene and cardiovascular events in osteoporotic postmenopausal women: four-year results from the MORE (Multiple Outcomes of Raloxifene Evaluation) randomized trial. *JAMA* 2002;**287**:847–57.

49. Yaffe K, Krueger K, Sarkar S et al. Cognitive function in postmenopausal women treated with raloxifene. *N Engl J Med* 2001;**344**:1207–13.

50. Bjarnason NH, Bjarnason K, Haarbo J et al. Tibolone: prevention of bone loss in late postmenopausal women. *J Clin Endocrinol Metab* 1996;**81**: 2419–22.

51. Berning B, Kuijk CV, Kuiper JW et al. Effects of two doses of tibolone on trabecular and cortical bone loss in early postmenopausal women: a two-year randomized, placebo-controlled study. *Bone* 1996;**19**:395–9.

52. Johannes EJ. Tibolone: vaginal bleeding and the specific endometrial response in postmenopausal women. *Gynecol Endocrinol* 1997;**11**(Suppl 2):25–30.

53. Fleisch H. *Bisphosphonates in Bone Disease: From the Laboratory to the Patient.* San Diego: Academic Press, 2000.

54. de Groen PC, Lubbe DF, Hirsch LJ et al. Esophagitis associated with the use of alendronate. *N Engl J Med* 1996;**335**:1016–21.

55. Storm T, Thamsborg G, Steiniche T et al. Effect of intermittent cyclical etidronate therapy on bone mass and fracture rate in women with postmenopausal osteoporosis. *N Engl J Med* 1990;**322**:1265–71.

56. Watts NB, Harris ST, Genant HK et al. Intermittent cyclical etidronate treatment of postmenopausal osteoporosis. *N Engl J Med* 1990;**323**:73–9.

57. Harris ST, Watts NB, Jackson RD et al. Four-year study of intermittent cyclic etidronate treatment of postmenopausal osteoporosis: three years of blinded therapy followed by one year of open therapy. *Am J Med* 1993;**95**:557–67.

58. Cranney A, Guyatt G, Krolicki N et al. A meta-analysis of etidronate for the treatment of postmenopausal osteoporosis. *Osteoporos Int* 2001;**12**: 140–51.

59. Hosking D, Chilvers CE, Christiansen C et al. Prevention of bone loss with alendronate in postmenopausal

women under 60 years of age. Early Postmenopausal Intervention Cohort Study Group. *N Engl J Med* 1998; **338**:485–92.

60. McClung M, Clemmesen B, Daifotis A et al. Alendronate prevents postmenopausal bone loss in women without osteoporosis. A double-blind, randomized, controlled trial. Alendronate Osteoporosis Prevention Study Group. *Ann Intern Med* 1998; **128**:253–61.

61. Black DM, Cummings SR, Karpf DB et al. Randomised trial of effect of alendronate on risk of fracture in women with existing vertebral fractures. Fracture Intervention Trial Research Group. *Lancet* 1996;**348**: 1535–41.

62. Cummings SR, Black DM, Thompson DE et al. Effect of alendronate on risk of fracture in women with low bone density but without vertebral fractures: results from the Fracture Intervention Trial. *JAMA* 1998;**280**: 2077–82.

63. Black DM, Thompson DE, Bauer DC et al. Fracture risk reduction with alendronate in women with osteoporosis: the Fracture Intervention Trial. FIT Research Group. *J Clin Endocrinol Metab* 2000;**85**:4118–24.

64. Pols HA, Felsenberg D, Hanley DA et al. Multinational, placebo-controlled, randomized trial of the effects of alendronate on bone density and fracture risk in postmenopausal women with low bone mass: results of the FOSIT study. Foxamax International Trial Study Group. *Osteoporos Int* 1999; **9**:461–8.

65. Tonino RP, Meunier PJ, Emkey R et al. Skeletal benefits of alendronate: 7-year treatment of postmenopausal osteoporotic women. Phase III Osteoporosis Treatment Study Group. *J Clin Endocrinol Metab* 2000;**85**:3109–15.

66. Schnitzer T, Bone HG, Crepaldi G et al. Therapeutic equivalence of alendronate 70 mg once-weekly and alendronate 10 mg daily in the treatment of osteoporosis. Alendronate Once-

Weekly Study Group. *Aging (Milano)* 2000;**12**:1–12.

67. Greenspan SL, Bone G 3rd, Schnitzer TJ et al. Two-year results of once-weekly administration of alendronate 70 mg for the treatment of postmenopausal osteoporosis. *J Bone Miner Res* 2002;**17**:1988–96.

68. Mortensen L, Charles P, Bekker PJ et al. Risedronate increases bone mass in an early postmenopausal population: two years of treatment plus one year of follow-up. *J Clin Endocrinol Metab* 1998;**83**:396–402.

69. Harris ST, Watts NB, Genant HK et al. Effects of risedronate treatment on vertebral and nonvertebral fractures in women with postmenopausal osteoporosis: a randomized controlled trial. Vertebral Efficacy With Risedronate Therapy (VERT) Study Group. *JAMA* 1999;**282**:1344–52.

70. Reginster J, Minne HW, Sorensen OH et al. Randomized trial of the effects of risedronate on vertebral fractures in women with established postmenopausal osteoporosis. Vertebral Efficacy with Risedronate Therapy (VERT) Study Group. *Osteoporos Int* 2000;**11**:83–91.

71. Sorensen OH, Crawford GM, Mulder H et al. Long-term efficacy of risedronate: a 5-year placebo-controlled clinical experience. *Bone* 2003;**32**: 120–6.

72. Watts NB, Josse RG, Hamdy RC et al. Risedronate prevents new vertebral fractures in postmenopausal women at high risk. *J Clin Endocrinol Metab* 2003;**88**:542–9.

73. Heaney RP, Zizic TM, Fogelman I et al. Risedronate reduces the risk of first vertebral fracture in osteoporotic women. *Osteoporos Int* 2002;**13**: 501–5.

74. McClung MR, Geusens P, Miller PD et al. Effect of risedronate on the risk of hip fracture in elderly women. Hip Intervention Program Study Group. *N Engl J Med* 2001;**344**:333–40.

75. McCloskey E, Selby P, de Takats D et al. Effects of clodronate on vertebral

fracture risk in osteoporosis: a 1-year interim analysis. *Bone* 2001;**28**: 310–15.

76. Lufkin EG, Argueta R, Whitaker MD et al. Pamidronate: an unrecognized problem in gastrointestinal tolerability. *Osteoporos Int* 1994;**4**:320–2.

77. Reid IR, Wattie DJ, Evans MC et al. Continuous therapy with pamidronate, a potent bisphosphonate, in postmenopausal osteoporosis. *J Clin Endocrinol Metab* 1994;**79**: 1595–9.

78. Reid IR, Brown JP, Burckhardt P et al. Intravenous zoledronic acid in postmenopausal women with low bone mineral density. *N Engl J Med* 2002; **346**:653–61.

79. Delmas PD, Recker RR, Stakkestad J et al. Oral ibandronate significantly reduces fracture risk in postmenopausal osteoporosis when administered daily or with a unique drug-free interval: Results from a pivotal phase III study. *Osteoporos Int* 2002;**13** (Suppl 1):S15.

80. Reginster JY, Deroisy R, Lecart MP et al. A double-blind, placebo-controlled, dose-finding trial of intermittent nasal salmon calcitonin for prevention of postmenopausal lumbar spine bone loss. *Am J Med* 1995;**98**:452–8.

81. Overgaard K, Riis BJ, Christiansen C, Hansen MA. Effect of salcatonin given intranasally on early postmenopausal bone loss. *BMJ* 1989;**299**:477–9.

82. Overgaard K, Hansen MA, Jensen SB, Christiansen C. Effect of salcatonin given intranasally on bone mass and fracture rates in established osteoporosis: a dose-response study. *BMJ* 1992;**305**:556–61.

83. Chesnut CH, 3rd, Silverman S, Andriano K et al. A randomized trial of nasal spray salmon calcitonin in postmenopausal women with established osteoporosis: the prevent recurrence of osteoporotic fractures study. PROOF Study Group. *Am J Med* 2000; **109**:267–76.

84. Seeman E, Delmas PD. Reconstructing the skeleton with intermittent parathyroid hormone. *Trends Endocrinol Metab* 2001;**12**:281–3.

85. Neer RM, Arnaud CD, Zanchetta JR et al. Effect of parathyroid hormone (1–34) on fractures and bone mineral density in postmenopausal women with osteoporosis. *N Engl J Med* 2001;**344**:1434–41.

86. Orimo H, Shiraki M, Hayashi T, Nakamura T. Reduced occurrence of vertebral crush fractures in senile osteoporosis treated with 1 alpha (OH)-vitamin D3. *Bone Miner* 1987;**3**: 47–52.

87. Orimo H, Shiraki M, Hayashi Y et al. Effects of 1 alpha-hydroxyvitamin D3 on lumbar bone mineral density and vertebral fractures in patients with postmenopausal osteoporosis. *Calcif Tissue Int* 1994;**54**:370–6.

88. Gallagher JC, Goldgar D. Treatment of postmenopausal osteoporosis with high doses of synthetic calcitriol. A randomized controlled study. *Ann Intern Med* 1990;**113**:649–55.

89. Gallagher JC, Riggs BL, Recker RR, Goldgar D. The effect of calcitriol on patients with postmenopausal osteoporosis with special reference to fracture frequency. *Proc Soc Exp Biol Med* 1989;**191**:287–92.

90. Tilyard MW, Spears GF, Thomson J, Dovey S. Treatment of postmenopausal osteoporosis with calcitriol or calcium. *N Engl J Med* 1992;**326**:357–62.

91. Meunier PJ, Sebert JL, Reginster JY et al. Fluoride salts are no better at preventing new vertebral fractures than calcium-vitamin D in postmenopausal osteoporosis: the FAVOS study. *Osteoporos Int* 1998;**8**:4–12.

92. Riggs BL, Hodgson SF, O'Fallon WM et al. Effect of fluoride treatment on the fracture rate in postmenopausal women with osteoporosis. *N Engl J Med* 1990;**322**:802–9.

93. Mamelle N, Meunier PJ, Dusan R et al. Risk-benefit ratio of sodium fluoride treatment in primary vertebral osteoporosis. *Lancet* 1988;**2**:361–5.

94. Szulc P, Chapuy MC, Meunier PJ, Delmas PD. Serum undercarboxylated osteocalcin is a marker of the risk of hip fracture in elderly women. *J Clin Invest* 1993;**91**:1769–74.

95. Orimo H, Shiraki M. Clinical evaluation of menatetrenone in the treatment of involutional osteoporosis. In: Christiansen C, Riis B, eds. *Proceedings* 1993. Fourth International Symposium on Osteoporosis, Hong Kong, 27 March – 2 April 1993: 148–9.

96. Shiraki M, Shiraki Y, Aoki C, Miura M. Vitamin K2 (menatetrenone) effectively prevents fractures and sustains lumbar bone mineral density in osteoporosis. *J Bone Miner Res* 2000;**15**: 515–21.

97. Marie PJ, Ammann P, Boivin G et al. Mechanisms of action and therapeutic potential of strontium in bone. *Calcif Tissue Int* 2001;**69**: 121–9.

98. Meunier PJ, Roux C, Seeman E et al. The effects of strontium ranelate on the risk of vertebral fracture in women with postmenopausal osteoporosis. *N Engl J Med* 2004;**350**: 459–68.

99. Rizzoli R, Reginster JY, Diaz Curiel M et al. Patients at high risk of hip fracture benefit from treatment with strontium ranelate. *Calc Tissue Int* 2004;**74**(Suppl 1):S83–4 (P152).

100. Alexandersen P, Toussaint A, Christiansen C et al. Ipriflavone in the treatment of postmenopausal osteoporosis: a randomized controlled trial. *JAMA* 2001;**285**:1482–8.

101. Mundy G, Garrett R, Harris S et al. Stimulation of bone formation in vitro and in rodents by statins. *Science* 1999;**286**:1946–9.

102. NIH Consensus Development Panel on Optimal Calcium Intake. *JAMA* 1994;**272**:1942–8.

103. Osteoporosis prevention, diagnosis, and therapy. *JAMA* 2001;**285**: 785–95.

104. Marcus R. The mechanism of exercise effects on bone. In: Bilezikian JP, Raisz LG, Rodan GA, eds. *Principles of Bone Biology*. San Diego: Academic Press, 1996:1435–45.

105. Fiatarone MA, Marks EC, Ryan ND et al. High-intensity strength training in nonagenarians. Effects on skeletal muscle. *JAMA* 1990;**263**: 3029–34.

106. Tinetti ME, Baker DI, McAvay G et al. A multifactorial intervention to reduce the risk of falling among elderly people living in the community. *N Engl J Med* 1994;**331**:821–7.

107. Taaffe DR, Duret C, Wheeler S, Marcus R. Once-weekly resistance exercise improves muscle strength and neuromuscular performance in older adults. *J Am Geriatr Soc* 1999; **47**:1208–14.

108. Lane JM, Girardi F, Parvataneni H et al. Preliminary outcomes of the first 226 consecutive kyphoplasties for the fixation of painful osteoporotic vertebral compression fractures. *Osteoporos Int* 2000;**11**(Suppl 2): S206.

109. Lauritzen JB, Petersen MM, Lund B. Effect of external hip protectors on hip fractures. *Lancet* 1993;**341**: 11–13.

110. Kannus P, Parkkari J, Niemi S et al. Prevention of hip fracture in elderly people with use of a hip protector. *N Engl J Med* 2000;**343**:1506–13.

111. Lindsay R, Silverman SL, Cooper C et al. Risk of new vertebral fracture in the year following a fracture. *JAMA* 2001;**285**:320–3.

112. Cummings SR, Palermo L, Browner W et al. Monitoring osteoporosis therapy with bone densitometry: misleading changes and regression to the mean. Fracture Intervention Trial Research Group. *JAMA* 2000; **283**:1318–21.

113. Garnero P, Shih WJ, Gineyts E et al. Comparison of new biochemical markers of bone turnover in late postmenopausal osteoporotic women in response to alendronate treatment. *J Clin Endocrinol Metab* 1994;**79**: 1693–700.

114. Ravn P, Christensen JO, Baumann M, Clemmesen B. Changes in biochemical markers and bone mass after withdrawal of ibandronate treatment: prediction of bone mass changes during treatment. *Bone* 1998;**22**:559–64.

115. Delmas PD, Hardy P, Garnero P, Dain M. Monitoring individual response to hormone replacement therapy with bone markers. *Bone* 2000;**26**: 553–60.

116. Delmas PD, Eastell R, Garnero P et al. The use of biochemical markers of bone turnover in osteoporosis. Committee of Scientific Advisors of the International Osteoporosis Foundation. *Osteoporos Int* 2000;**11**(Suppl 6):S2–S17.

117. Bjarnason NH, Sarkar S, Duong T et al. Six and twelve month changes in bone turnover are related to reduction in vertebral fracture risk during 3 years of raloxifene treatment in postmenopausal osteoporosis. *Osteoporos Int* 2001;**12**:922–30.

118. Eastell R, Barton I, Hannon RA et al. Relationship of early changes in bone resorption to the reduction in fracture risk with risedronate. *J Bone Miner Res* 2003;**18**:1051–6.

119. Riggs BL, Melton LJ 3rd, O'Fallon WM. Drug therapy for vertebral fractures in osteoporosis: evidence that decreases in bone turnover and increases in bone mass both determine antifracture efficacy. *Bone* 1996 **18**(Suppl 3):S197–S201.

120. Liberman UA, Weiss SR, Broll J et al. Effect of oral alendronate on bone mineral density and the incidence of fractures in postmenopausal osteoporosis. The Alendronate Phase III Osteoporosis Treatment Study Group. *N Engl J Med* 1995;**333**: 1437–43.

121. Boivin GY, Chavassieux PM, Santora AC et al. Alendronate increases bone strength by increasing the mean degree of mineralization of bone tissue in osteoporotic women. *Bone* 2000;**27**:687–94.

122. Delmas PD. How does antiresorptive therapy decrease the risk of fracture in women with osteoporosis? *Bone* 2000;**27**:1–3.

123. Lindsay R, Nieves J, Formica C et al. Randomised controlled study of effect of parathyroid hormone on vertebral-bone mass and fracture incidence among postmenopausal women on oestrogen with osteoporosis. *Lancet* 1997;**350**: 550–5.

124. Delmas PD, Calvo G, Boers M et al. The use of placebo-controlled and non-inferiority trials for the evaluation of new drugs in the treatment of postmenopausal osteoporosis. *Osteoporos Int* 2002;**13**:1–5.

125. Delmas PD. Treatment of postmenopausal osteoporosis. *Lancet* 2002;**359**:2018–26.

6
Economic aspects of osteoporosis

Rachael L Fleurence, Cynthia P Iglesias and David J Torgerson

INTRODUCTION

Fragility fractures as a consequence of osteoporosis are a major public health problem. This disease burden will increase due to an ageing population. The outcomes of fractures are widespread, and include an increase in health care expenditure as well as a rise in morbidity and mortality due to the disease.

Whilst the cost and health impact of osteoporosis have been well documented, of greater importance is how fractures should be prevented and at what cost. This chapter considers the cost-effectiveness of the most widely used treatments for fracture prevention. The chapter is based upon a review that two of the authors (RLF, CPI) have undertaken of all the published economic evaluations of treatments for osteoporosis.

However, before we assess the efficiency of various treatments we will first briefly consider the main evaluative methods economists use to assess whether a treatment is likely to give good value for money or not.

ECONOMIC EVALUATION METHODS

The purpose of economic evaluations is to help decision-makers determine whether the extra cost of an intervention that is more effective than current practice, can be justified given the limited resources available for health care programmes. In the UK, it is generally assumed that cost-effective interventions are valued between £10,000 and £30,000 per quality adjusted life year (QALY).[1] However, there is no agreed upper limit separating cost-effective interventions from others. The following section briefly outlines the three different types of economic evaluations: cost-effectiveness, cost-utility and cost-benefit analyses.[2]

Cost-effectiveness

A cost-effectiveness analysis compares the differences in costs and effectiveness of two or more interventions. In this type of economic evaluation, effectiveness is measured in natural units. In the field of osteoporosis prevention, possible natural units are the number of fractures avoided or the QALY scores obtained using specific instruments from fracture patients. Obviously, cost-effectiveness studies can only provide information on interventions measured in the same units. Thus, cost-effectiveness analyses can usefully compare different interventions aimed at preventing osteoporosis, but such analyses would not help to determine whether these interventions were cost-effective compared to a treatment for heart disease, for example. One way to overcome this shortcoming is to use life years gained as the measure of effectiveness, which allows for comparisons across diseases. However, the use of life years gained would not account for the impact on quality of life of the treatment. In determining which type of economic evaluation is best suited to the intervention under consideration, it is important to determine beforehand whether the impact of mortality is sufficient or whether QALY considerations should also be included.

Costs to be accounted for in an economic evaluation should ideally include all costs incurred by society, ranging from the health service costs to the out-of-pocket payments made by the patient and losses of productivity due to the condition. However, in practice, few economic evaluations include indirect costs and many tend to adopt the perspective of the health system. This may underestimate the cost-effectiveness of a treatment for the prevention of osteoporosis if these are associated with time lost from work. Some issues remain unresolved on the question of whether future costs incurred due to increased life expectancy should be included.[3] In the case of treatments to prevent osteoporosis, the costs of treatments and any costs incurred by the health service from side effects of the treatment would need to be included. The issues surrounding the calculation and the nature of costs are the same for the three types of analysis.

Cost-utility

Probably the most useful technique for assessing the economic value of treatments for the prevention of osteoporosis is cost-utility analysis. A cost-utility analysis compares the costs and the utilities of two or more interventions. A utility is the measure of the preference or value placed upon a health state and is a number between 0 (representing death) and 1 (perfect health); so, for example, a woman with a hip fracture may value her present quality of life at 0.7. If she suffered the hip fracture 10 years ago, she will have lived 7 QALYs compared to a women in perfect health for 10 years, who will have lived 10 QALYs.

The issue of who should evaluate health states is still unresolved, yet this is an important issue, because different sources can provide widely varying utilities.[4] In practice, these values are generally elicited from the patients but sometimes have to be determined by health professionals or significant family members. Several methods have been proposed to elicit these utility values. The simplest is the rating scale method, which asks the respondent to mark on a straight line with grid marks, a number corresponding to her perceived quality of life. However, economic theory would suggest that this method is the weakest in terms of deriving an estimate of the true utility value of a respondent. Theoretically superior, but more difficult for the respondent to understand, are the standard gamble and the time trade-off methods. These techniques elicit utility preferences from respondents by presenting them with successive choices between health states (or time spent in health states) to which different probabilities are attached. Other methods to calculate utilities use generic health state questionnaires, such as the Euroqol or the Health State Utilities Index, that provide utilities for health states on the basis of the responses of the subject.[2] Once these utilities have been obtained, it is possible to calculate QALYs.

One of the advantages of using QALYs is that they allow for comparisons between interventions across different conditions, so unlike cost-effectiveness studies, a comparison between a treatment for heart disease and a preventive treatment for osteoporosis can be done. By using QALYs, it is possible to evaluate interventions that impact on the quality as well as the length of life. For example, in studies looking at HRT, benefits, such as reduction in fracture risk and alleviation of menopausal symptoms, can be incorporated alongside potential risks, such as breast cancer or endometrial cancer.

Cost-benefit

A cost-benefit evaluation explicitly places a monetary valuation on the outcomes of health care and seeks to determine whether a health technology provides an overall net gain to society, in the sense where the benefits outweigh the costs. So, for example, a cost-benefit analysis would seek to put a monetary value on the number of hip fractures avoided, or the number of QALYs gained through the implementation of a preventive program. Several approaches have been used in cost-benefit analyses in health care, although many problems remain in practice.[5] Nonetheless, recently there has been considerable interest in techniques, such as contingent valuation, which elicit monetary valuations by asking people for their stated preferences among specified choices in monetary terms. This so-called 'willingness to pay' approach asks people how much they would be prepared to pay to obtain the benefits of an intervention or avoid the costs of illness. Applications of cost-benefit analyses in health care have been relatively rare, partly due to the difficulty in eliciting reliable 'willingness to pay' measures and partly due to the resistance, particularly amongst health professionals, in placing a monetary valuation on health benefits.

Addressing uncertainty

The purpose of economic evaluations is to inform decision-making by helping to make rational choices between different intervention strategies. However, in a number of cases decision-makers will have to make choices without necessarily having robust data on long-term effectiveness and cost-effectiveness of the interventions under consideration. Indeed, a number of parameters influencing the final decision will be uncertain, ranging from the costs of treatments and interventions to the effectiveness of the interventions under consideration. Addressing the uncertainty in economic evaluations should constitute an essential component of the analysis.[6,7] Several methods have been proposed to tackle uncertainty in cost-effectiveness analyses. One-way sensitivity analyses vary a specific parameter within a plausible range and assess the impact of this variation on the results of the economic evaluation. One-way sensitivity analysis however remains quite limited in that it can only account for variations in one parameter at a time and cannot account for interactions between parameters. Multi-way sensitivity analysis can overcome some of the drawbacks of one-way sensitivity analysis by varying several parameters simultaneously. However, this method becomes quickly unmanageable when the number of parameters is important and the results are difficult to represent in a succinct manner. Probabilistic sensitivity analysis on the other hand can account for the joint variation of parameters in an economic evaluation. Each input parameter is assigned an appropriate statistical distribution and a 95% confidence interval, representing a range of plausible values that are obtained from the literature.[8] A Monte-Carlo simulation is then run to obtain a large number of iterations of the model. A succinct way of representing the results of the probabilistic sensitivity analysis is to use cost-effectiveness acceptability curves.[8,9] These graphs show the probability that an intervention is cost-effective as a function of the decision-maker's ceiling cost-effectiveness ratio (this ceiling will vary according to the resources available for health care and is in general unknown to the analyst).[9,10]

For example, Iglesias et al (2002) described the uncertainty around the cost-effectiveness of risedronate using confidence intervals.[11] An alternative approach would have been to use a cost-effectiveness acceptability curve (CEAC). Using data generated for the economic model of risedronate the CEAC of risedronate can be shown (see Figure 6.1). The cost-effectiveness acceptability curve of risedronate versus placebo is presented for women aged 75 years who had experienced a previous vertebral fracture. According to this analysis the probability of risedronate being cost-effective assuming a decision-maker's willingness to pay for a hip fracture averted of £10,000 is 99.3%, for values above £10,000 the probability of risedronate being cost-effective is almost 100%.

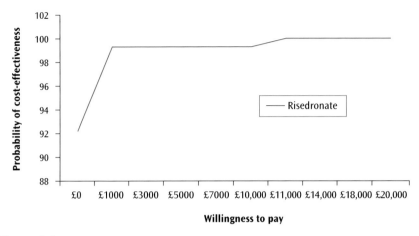

Figure 6.1
Cost-effective acceptability curve (CEAC) of risedronate.

COST-EFFECTIVENESS OF TREATMENTS FOR FRACTURE PREVENTION

There are an increasing number of effective methods for preventing fragility fractures. Many of these therapies have been shown to be effective in large, rigorously designed, randomized controlled trials: the gold standard for evidence-based medicine. In this section we will consider the effectiveness and cost-effectiveness of some of the more widely used interventions.

HORMONAL TREATMENTS

Estrogen replacement therapy

Hormone replacement therapy (HRT), traditionally, was seen as the gold-standard therapy for the treatment and prevention of postmenopausal osteoporosis.[12] Observational data consistently show that HRT use is associated with a reduction in fractures. Furthermore, meta-analyses of randomized trials also show a beneficial effect on the occurrence of fractures. Two meta-analyses by Torgerson and Bell-Syer noted a 27% reduction and 33% reduction in all nonvertebral and vertebral fractures, respectively, through the use of HRT.[13,14] Including data from trials published since still showed a statistically significant 20% reduction in all fractures.[15]

The publication of the Women's Health Initiative (WHI) trial has confirmed the meta-analyses of randomized data as to the benefit of HRT on fractures. The WHI study showed an approximate reduction of 24% and 34% in all fractures and hip fractures, respectively.[16] In Figure 6.2 we update the HRT meta-analyses on all fractures. As the analysis shows HRT is still associated with a highly statistically significant reduction in all fractures. However, in economic models the use of HRT for osteoporosis prevention is driven, not by its effects on fractures but for its other effects.

A systematic review of all economic evaluations by Torgerson and Reid in 1997 concluded that the cost effectiveness of HRT is dominated by its effects on the cardiovascular system.[17] If HRT did reduce cardiovascular events by

Comparison: 01 HRT vs control
Outcome: 01 HRT vs control

Study	HRT n/N	Control n/N	RR (95%CI Random)	Weight %	RR (95%CI Random)
Aitkin	0/68	2/66		0.2	0.19[0.01,3.97]
Alexandersen	2/51	6/49		0.9	0.32[0.07,1.51]
Bjarnson	4/112	1/41		0.5	1.46[0.17,12.72]
Bone	18/283	9/142		3.3	1.00[0.46,2.18]
Cheng	1/40	1/40		0.3	1.00[0.06,15.44]
Delmas	1/90	2/45		0.4	0.25[0.02,2.68]
Eiken	1/100	6/51		0.5	0.08[0.01,0.69]
Eli Lilly	12/158	3/152		1.4	3.85[1.11,13.37]
Gallagher	24/243	19/246		5.6	1.28[0.72,2.27]
Genant	3/303	2/103		0.7	0.51[0.09,3.01]
HERs	138/1370	148/1383		20.0	0.94[0.76,1.17]
Herrington	13/204	15/105		3.9	0.45[0.22,0.90]
Ishida	0/30	3/30		0.3	0.14[0.01,2.65]
Komulainen	13/232	27/232		4.7	0.48[0.25,0.91]
Lees	10/466	3/113		1.3	0.81[0.23,2.89]
Lindsay	1/25	2/25		0.4	0.50[0.05,5.17]
Mosekilde	33/502	43/504		8.7	0.77[0.50,1.19]
Mulnard	1/81	0/39		0.2	1.46[0.06,35.13]
Nachtigall	0/84	6/84		0.3	0.08[0.00,1.34]
Orr-Walker	2/11	1/12		0.4	2.18[0.23,20.84]
PEPI	21/701	6/174		2.6	0.87[0.36,2.12]
Ravn	5/110	39/502		2.5	0.59[0.24,1.45]
Recker	7/64	6/64		1.9	1.17[0.41,3.28]
Viscoli	30/337	33/327		7.8	0.88[0.55,1.41]
WHI	650/8506	788/8102		30.7	0.79[0.71,0.87]
Weiss	3/129	1/46		0.4	1.07[0.11,10.03]
Wimalawansa	1/18	1/18		0.3	1.00[0.07,14.79]
Total(95%CI)	994/14318	1173/12695		100.0	0.81[0.70,0.94]

Test for heterogeneity chi-square=30.67 df=26 p=0.24
Test for overall effect z − 2.83 p=0.005

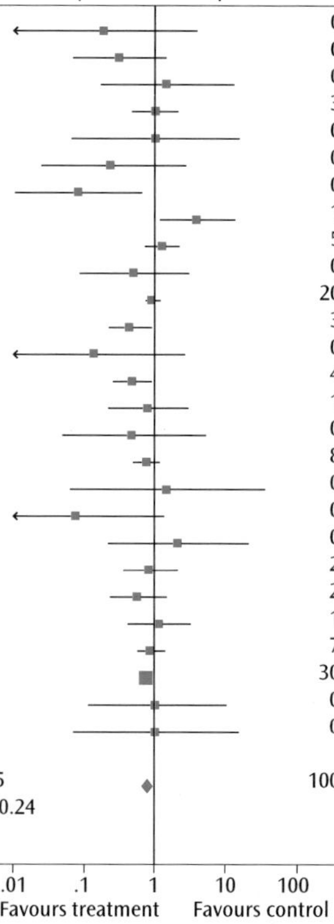

.01   .1   1   10   100
Favours treatment   Favours control

Figure 6.2

HRT meta-analyses on all fractures.

around 50%, as indicated by observational data, and its effects on breast cancer incidence was modest, then long-term treatment of women at low or average risk of fracture seemed a relatively cost-effective option. Within the last five years the view of HRT preventing cardiovascular events has substantially changed. First, the publication of the HER trial of HRT for the secondary prevention of cardiovascular disease noted an *increase* in cardiovascular events.[18] Second, the early termination and publication of the WHI trial in 2002 because of an increase in cardiovascular events confirmed that HRT was hazardous to the cardiovascular system.[16] Along with an increased incidence of breast cancer, then the view that HRT would be a cost-effective long-term preventive measure for osteoporosis is no longer tenable. Nevertheless, among women with no predisposing risk factors for cardiovascular disease the absolute risk of sustaining a cardiovascular event as a consequence of using HRT is relatively slight. HRT may be still a relatively cost-effective method of fracture prevention among women with a high risk of fracture with an average or lower risk of cardiovascular disease. For example, women who have had an early menopause or hysterectomy have an elevated risk of fracture as do women who have low body weight, with the latter group being at reduced risk of cardiovascular disease. For these groups of women HRT might, in some circumstances, be a cost-effective option for fracture prevention. For example, women aged between 55 and 59 years who have three fracture risk factors (i.e. early menopause plus already sustained 2 fractures) will have an absolute risk of fracture of about 9%.[19] For these women HRT is a relatively inexpensive treatment option and because their absolute risk of fracture is many times that of their risk of cardiovascular disease or breast cancer then the benefits of treatment may outweigh the disadvantages. Treating women with such a high absolute risk of fracture may be relatively cost-effective with a simple modelling exercise indicating that treatment with the cheapest unopposed estrogen (appropriate for women with a prior hysterectomy) led to a cost per averted fracture of less than £1000.[19] Indeed, the most recently published WHI study of estrogens alone suggests that when women who have had a hysterectomy are given unopposed estrogens, there may be a slight reduction in breast cancer and no detrimental effect on coronary heart disease.[20] These data suggest that estrogen-alone therapy for hysterectomized women could be cost effective.

Fleurence et al (2002) in the only economic analysis published to date that used patient specific data suggested that for women aged around 55 years who had had a prior hysterectomy the cost per averted fracture was less than £2000.[12] Whether these cost-effectiveness ratios are 'worthwhile' will depend upon a decision-maker's 'willingness to pay' for the prevention of a fracture. For women aged between 50 and 60 years the majority of fractures that would be prevented are relatively 'minor' fractures such as Colles' and digital fractures. Incident hip fractures among such a population are exceedingly rare. The Fleurence study is also the only published economic evaluation to use CEACs, which are reproduced in Figures 6.3a and 6.3b.

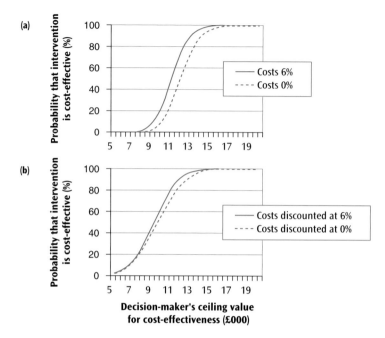

Figure 6.3

Cost-effectiveness acceptability curves (CEAC); (a) HRT in the general population; (b) HRT in the high-risk population. Source: Reproduced with permission of Springer-Verlag London Ltd, from Fleurence et al[12].)

BISPHOSPHONATES

Bisphosphonates have been shown to reduce hip fractures in randomized trials. In particular, for alendronate and risedronate there are large trials in which their use has been associated with significant reductions in hip fractures. In a trial powered to detect reductions in hip fractures risedronate was associated with a 60% reduction of hip fractures in women aged 70–79 years, and with a previous vertebral fracture.[21] Alendronate was associated with a 49% reduction in a similar cohort of patients.[22,23] However, according to the results of a meta-analysis a third bisphosphonate available in the UK, etidronate, was recently deemed as ineffective at preventing nonvertebral fractures.[24]

Whilst there have been large *effectiveness* trials of bisphosphonates their cost-effectiveness has been ascertained using model based evaluations as cost data were not routinely collected as part of the trial. The cost-effectiveness of bisphosphonates in the treatment of osteoporotic patients has been investigated using decision analytic models. At least five different models investigating the cost-effectiveness of bisphosphonate therapies were identified.[11,25–28] A summary of these studies are described in Table 6.1.

Markov models and simple decision trees have been the preferred option to describe the prognosis of patients with osteoporosis. Individuals represented in the models are usually those who are considered to be at a higher risk of fractures (i.e. postmenopausal women aged 75 years or over who have been previously diagnosed with a vertebral fracture).

In all but one of the identified studies the health benefit associated with bisphosphonate therapies was measured in terms of the number of hip fractures averted. Francis et al defined the number of vertebral fractures prevented as the measure of benefit for their economic analysis.[26] The selection of number of hip fractures averted as a meaningful health outcome measure for an economic analysis has been mainly justified on the higher costs associated with the treatment of this type of fracture in comparison to the costs of treating the other two most common osteoporotic fractures, vertebral and wrist fractures. Whilst the impact on an individual's quality of life associated with osteoporotic fractures has been frequently discussed in the literature, however in only one study QALYs were used as an alternative measure of health benefit.[11]

No head-to-head comparisons of the different therapies for the treatment of osteoporosis are available, consequently placebo therapy has invariably been the comparator chosen in the economic analyses. The size of the health benefit associated with bisphosphonate therapies in the different modelling exercises is based on the 'best' available published evidence at the time when each of the economic analyses were conducted.

The estimation of costs per fracture in all the analyses concentrated only on the estimation of direct costs associated with different types of fractures; hip, vertebral and wrist, from the perspective of a health services provider. Items usually included in costing were pharmaceutical therapy costs, and cost of fracture; which mainly included GP visits, hospital cost, and physiotherapy costs. Indirect costs associated with the sequels of osteoporotic fractures have not been included in any of the existing modelling exercises.

According to all but one of the modeling exercises bisphosphonates have been identified as a potentially cost-effective intervention for the prevention of hip fractures. In a Spanish study, alendronate was identified as a non cost-effective intervention.[27]

Four out of the five identified models were deterministic (i.e. the uncertainty surrounding the point estimates of the different parameters within the models was not characterized). In other words, model parameters were defined as single values. Only one of the models was stochastic, in which probability distribution functions were associated to all stochastic parameters within the model.[11] Monte-Carlo simulations were used to propagate probability distributions. The results of this analysis have been presented following the most conventionally used cost-effectiveness ratios and the uncertainty surrounding such estimates was represented using non-parametric methods to estimate 95% confidence intervals (CI).

Table 6.1 Economic evaluation studies of bisphosphonate therapies for the prevention of osteoporotic fractures

Study	Intervention	Control	Population	Health benefit	Costs	Incremental analysis	Sensitivity analysis	Conclusions
Francis, 1988[26] UK	HRT, etidronate, salmon calcitonin	Placebo	Post-menopausal women with vertebral established osteoporosis	*Vertebral fractures (VFx) averted.* HRT and calcitonin 60% reduction of VF. Etidronate 53% to 58% reduction of VFx.	*Cost per fracture avoided* Calcitonin: £9075–£25,013 HRT: £138–£680 Etidronate: £1880	Not performed	Not performed	VFx may be averted at relatively low cost with etidronate and HRT.
Ankjaer-Jensen, 1996[25] Denmark	Calcium, etidronate, calcitonin, (5 years) and HRT (10 years)	Placebo	Danish healthy women aged 70 years	*Hip fractures (HFx) averted.* Two scenarios: optimistic and pessimistic. Fracture Relative Risk (RR) for calcitonin, etidronate, calcium and HRT was 0.23, 0.5, 0.5, and 0.5 for the optimistic scenario. RR for calcitonin, etidronate, calcium and HRT was 0.70, 0.5, 0.75, and 0.75 for the pessimistic scenario.	*Cost per fracture avoided* 142,300 DDK, –10,864 DDK, 7609 DDK, –38,909 DDK, and 6018 DDK for calcitonin, etidronate, calcium, HRT pills and HRT patch, respectively.	Not performed	Results sensitive to changes in HFx costs.	There are large differences in the cost-effectiveness of different pharmaceutical treatments. Etidronate has the lowest cost-effectiveness ratio and calcitonin the highest.

Study	Intervention	Control	Population	Health benefit	Costs	Incremental analysis	Sensitivity analysis	Conclusions
Visentin, 1997[28] Italy	Calcitonin, bisphosphonates (clodronate, etidronate, alendronate), HRT, Vitamin D (1-year treatment)	Placebo	Italian women over 50 years	*Hip fractures averted* All drugs were associated with a 33% reduction in fracture.	*Cost per fracture averted* $1.6, $0.06, $0.1, $0.2 million per fracture averted were associated with calcitonin, HRT, bisphosphonates and vitamin D	Not performed	Not performed	HRT seems to be the best option for the prevention of hip fractures.
Rodriguez, 1999[27] Spain	Alendronate	Placebo	Spanish women with established osteoporosis	*Hip fractures averted* A hip fracture reduction of 51% was assumed.	*Cost per fracture averted* Cost per fracture averted of 297.9 and 23.3 thousand pesetas were associated with alendronate and placebo, respectively.	ICER per averted fracture was 25.6 million pesetas.	Model was sensitive to changes in the clinical effectiveness associated with alendronate.	Given the current price of alendronate in Spain this is not a cost-effective therapy for the prevention of hip fractures.
Iglesias, 2002[11] UK	3-year risedronate therapy	Placebo	75-year-old British women	*Hip, vertebral, and other (wrist) fractures averted* Fracture reductions of 60%, 41% and 39% were assumed for hip, vertebral and other fractures, respectively QALYs gained per patient 0.043.	*Cost per fracture averted* Costs per fracture averted were £786.	Dominant therapy	The model was sensitive to changes in the follow-up period, and changes in the incidence of hip fractures.	Risedronate is a dominant treatment for women aged >75 with low bone mineral density and a prior vertebral fracture.

ICER = incremental cost-effectiveness ratio.

CALCIUM WITH VITAMIN D

There is some evidence that vitamin D with calcium supplementation has a positive effect in decreasing fracture rates. In a clinical trial of daily supplements of oral vitamin D_3 with calcium, Chapuy et al (1992) showed that in elderly women, hip fracture rates decreased by 26%.[29] Dawson-Hughes et al (1997) showed that calcium and vitamin D supplementation in men and women over 65 years old decreased the number of nonvertebral fractures by 54%.[30] Whether vitamin D alone is also effective is still under question. Heikinheimo et al reported that fracture rates decreased in elderly patients given a vitamin D injection, although this trial may not have been appropriately randomized.[31] However, in a clinical trial of oral vitamin D alone, Lips et al found no significant difference between the intervention and control groups.[32]

From a public health perspective, decision-makers need to choose between strategies for the prevention of osteoporosis that will be the most beneficial for patients, while taking into account the limited resources available for such programs. Because of the relative low cost of vitamin supplements compared to other available treatments for osteoporosis, such as HRT and bisphosphonates, establishing the cost-effectiveness of strategies involving nutritional supplements is likely to be an essential step in the overall decision process of putting prevention strategies into practice.

Economic evaluations: vitamin D with calcium

A review of the literature found six published economic evaluations analysing the cost-effectiveness of strategies involving vitamin D with or without calcium supplementation.[25,27,33–36] To date, no economic evaluations of supplements have been based on clinical data, so that all evaluations used some form of modelling to explore the cost-effectiveness of the strategies. The following section summarizes each study briefly. Detailed results of the evaluations are reported in Table 6.2.

Geelhoed et al (1994) analysed a number of strategies with estrogen replacement therapy, calcium and exercise, compared to no intervention in healthy Caucasian women aged 50 years onwards.[37] The perspective of the study was the Australian Health Service. The main source of the clinical data was an assumption, based on the authors' judgment, that calcium halved the rate of bone loss without treatment. The main source of the cost data was the hospital in which the study took place. The authors found that lifetime estrogen therapy from age 50 years onwards was the most cost-effective treatment.

Torgerson and Kanis (1995) compared vitamin D by injection and vitamin D and calcium to no preventive strategy, in women with and without low body mass index (BMI), in women living in the community and in institutional settings.[34] The perspective of the analysis was the UK National Health Service. The main source of the clinical data was the literature, including one

Table 6.2 Economic evaluation studies of vitamin D and calcium for the prevention of osteoporotic fractures

Study	Intervention	Control	Population	Health benefits	Cost-effectiveness results*	Sensitivity analysis	Cost-effectiveness conclusions
Geelhoed, 1994[33]	Different strategies with HRT, calcium, and exercise	No intervention	Healthy Caucasian women from age 50 years onwards	The number of QALYs per women was 32 for no intervention, between 32 and 33 for HRT regimens, and 32 for calcium and exercise.	The cost per QALY gained was between $8500 and $16,500 for HRT regimens and $28,500 for calcium and exercise.	Results were sensitive to assumptions about the cardio-protective effects of HRT, nursing home costs, and risk of breast cancer.	Lifetime HRT from age 50 years was the most cost-effective treatment.
Torgerson, 1995[34]	VD by injection and VDC	No intervention	Women with and without low BMI in community and institutional settings	VD injection: all fractures ↓ 25%, hip fractures ↓ 22%. Oral VDC: all fractures ↓ 21%, hip fractures ↓ 28%.	Net cost per averted hip fracture ranged from −£2221 to £17,379 for VD injection and from: £4781 to −£2573 for VDC.	Not performed	VD injection is potentially cost-effective in the elderly population. VDC may be cost-effective in targeted high-risk populations.

Table 6.2 continued

Study	Intervention	Control	Population	Health benefits	Cost-effectiveness results*	Sensitivity analysis	Cost-effectiveness conclusions
Torgerson, 1996[36]	VD by injection, thiazide, HRT, VDC, calcium, and calcitonin	No intervention	Hypothetical cohort of women aged 80 years	The number of hip fractures avoided for VD injection, thiazide, HRT, calcium, and calcitonin was 1867, 1527, 2546, 2291, 1527, and 3140, respectively.	ICERs (including averted costs) were a cost-saving of £9,176,496 for VD injection, a cost-saving of £4,775,704 for thiazide (compared to do-nothing), £41,493 for HRT, £81,547 for VDC, and £433,548 for calcitonin. Calcium was dominated.	Results were sensitive to the assumptions about the effectiveness of treatments.	The study concluded that VD was potentially the most cost-effective treatment, given the assumptions of the model. Further research into the effectiveness of VD and VDC should be conducted.

Study	Intervention	Control	Population	Health benefits	Cost-effectiveness results*	Sensitivity analysis	Cost-effectiveness conclusions
Ankjaer-Jensen, 1996[25]	Calcium, etidronate, and calcitonin for 5 years, HRT for 10 years	No intervention	Women aged 70 years at onset of treatment and women screened for low BMD	For all women over 70, under *optimistic* assumptions, the number of hip fractures avoided was 0.17 with calcitonin, 0.11 with etidronate, 0.11 with calcium, and 0.11 with HRT. Under *pessimistic* assumptions, the number of hip fractures avoided was 0.04 with calcitonin, 0.07 with etidronate, 0.03 with calcium, and 0.03 with HRT.	The cost-effectiveness ratio ranged from 140,000 to 860,000 DKK for calcitonin, from 10,864 to 24,400 for etidronate, from 7600 to 220,000 for calcium and from cost-saving to 178,000 for HRT, depending on *optimistic* and *pessimistic* assumptions.	*Optimistic* and *pessimistic* scenarios were used.	Etidronate has the lowest cost-effectiveness ratio and calcitonin has the highest. [Reviewer's note: because of methodological problems in this study, conclusions should be viewed with caution].
Rodriguez, 1999[27]	Alendronate	VDC	Women with established osteoporosis and a previous vertebral fracture	1.1% of women taking alendronate had a hip fracture, compared to 2.2 % taking VDC.	Incremental cost per fracture averted was 25.6 million pesetas.	Model was sensitive to changes in the clinical effectiveness associated with alendronate.	Alendronate is not a cost-effective intervention.

Table 6.2 continued

Study	Intervention	Control	Population	Health benefits	Cost-effectiveness results*	Sensitivity analysis	Cost-effectiveness conclusions
Bendich, 1999[35]	Daily calcium supplementation	No intervention	Individuals aged 50+ in the USA	Daily intake of calcium would prevent 134,764 hip fractures in individuals aged 50+ in the USA	Not calculated	Results were sensitive to cost of hip fractures, duration and cost of supplements, pre-existing use of supplements alone or in conjunction with estrogen or bisphosphonates	Calcium is cost-effective for women aged 75+ years and possibly for all individuals aged 65+ years

* Negative cost-effectiveness ratios indicate cost-saving according to the authors, however, there are methodological problems in interpreting negative cost-effectiveness ratios and they should be used with caution.

BMD, bone mineral density; BMI, body mass index; ICER, incremental cost-effectiveness ratio; VD, vitamin D; VDC, oral vitamin D and calcium.

randomized controlled trial and two observational studies. Costs were obtained from published sources and NHS fees. The study concluded that vitamin D injection was potentially cost-effective in the elderly population and that vitamin D and calcium may be cost-effective in targeted high risk populations. However, since that study was undertaken the cost of calcium and vitamin D supplements, in the UK, have fallen substantially, which makes their use more cost-effective among a lower risk population.

Torgerson et al (1996) analysed vitamin D injection, thiazide, HRT, vitamin D and calcium and calcitonin in a hypothetical cohort of women aged 80.[36] The perspective was the UK National Health Service. The source of the clinical data was 2 randomized trials, 2 case-control studies and 1 meta-analysis of observational studies. The source of the cost data was published prices in the UK. The study concluded that vitamin D was potentially the most cost-effective treatment, and that further research into the effectiveness of vitamin D and vitamin D and calcium should be conducted. This finding is given further support with the recent publication of a trial of oral vitamin D supplementation, which noted a significant reduction in nonvertebral fractures among, mainly, retired doctors.[38]

Ankjaer-Jensen et al (1996) investigated calcium, etidronate and calcitonin for 5 years and HRT for 10 years in women aged 70 and in women screened for low bone density measurement (BDM).[25] The perspective of the study was the Danish health system. The main source of the clinical data was three published studies. The source of the cost data was not reported in detail. The authors concluded that etidronate had the lowest cost-effectiveness ratio and calcitonin had the highest.

Rodriguez et al (1999) compared alendronate to vitamin D and calcium in women with established osteoporosis.[27] The perspective of the study was the Spanish health system. The clinical data was obtained from previously published studies. Spanish hospital and drug prices were used in the costing. The study concluded that alendronate was not a cost-effective intervention.

Bendich et al (1999) examined the cost-effectiveness of daily calcium supplementation in individuals over 50 years in the USA.[35] The perspective was that of society (USA). The source of the clinical data was three randomized controlled trials. The costing data was obtained from published US sources. The study concluded that calcium was cost-effective for women aged 75 years and more and possible for all individuals aged 65 years and more.

Economic evaluations: validity of results

While economic evaluations constitute invaluable tools for resource allocation decisions, the quality and validity of these studies must be established before they can be used by decision-makers. For example, in terms of the quality of the clinical data used in the evaluations of vitamin D and calcium, only Torgerson et al (1995, 1996) used the most recent evidence and described in detail the original clinical studies that were used for the analysis.[34,36] In contrast,

Geelhoed et al (1994) used now out-of-date assumptions concerning the cardio-protective effect of HRT, and Rodriguez et al (1999) and Ankjaer-Jensen (1996) do not report in detail the rationale for selecting the studies used in their analysis.[25,27,33] Finally, Bendich used trial results for vitamin D and calcium, although the analysis was purportedly looking at calcium supplementation alone.[35] Another criteria to look for when assessing the quality of economic evaluations, is how appropriately the rules of cost-effectiveness analysis were applied. Indeed there are definite methodological concerns in the studies by Ankjaer-Jensen (1996) and by Geelhoed et al (1994), while the study by Bendich et al (1999) does not technically constitute a cost-effectiveness study but rather a calculation of total cost savings and total hip fractures avoided.[25,33,35] However, both studies by Torgerson (1995, 1996) and the study by Rodriguez (1999) apply the rules correctly.[27,34,36] Finally a useful part of the economic evaluation is the sensitivity analysis. All six studies use one- or multi-way sensitivity analysis, if at all, which as discussed in the above section on handling uncertainty, is less useful than probabilistic sensitivity analysis, because it cannot appropriately account for the joint variation of parameters within the analysis.

In conclusion, caution is advised when using these economic evaluations because of the uneven quality of the studies. In particular, the results of the studies by Geelhoed et al (1994), Ankjaer-Jensen (1996), Rodriguez et al (1999) and Bendich et al (1999) should be viewed with some caution.[25,27,33,35] Based on the two studies by Torgerson et al (1995, 1996), current evidence indicates that vitamin D with or without calcium supplementation is probably cost-effective in the UK, in particular in high risk groups such as older women and women who have previously sustained fractures.[34,36] However, stronger evidence on the effectiveness of both treatments is still needed.

TARGETING TREATMENTS

One of the key drivers of an economic evaluation is the absolute incidence of fracture. All things being equal, treating a population with a high fracture incidence is likely to be more cost-effective than treating one with a low fracture incidence. Epidemiological studies have highlighted a number of important risk factors for fracture. The strongest single predictor of fracture risk is low bone mineral density (BMD). There are other important predictors of fracture risk. The strongest epidemiological evidence for fracture risk comes from the Study of Osteoporotic Fractures (SOFt). In this study of nearly 10,000 Caucasian women aged 65 years and over a range of important predictors of fracture risk were established.[39]

Low body weight, particularly body weight of less than 58 kg is an important risk factor for fracture. This risk factor, however, is strongly correlated with BMD and when bone mass measurements are available it is of only minor importance. In contrast, other risk factors remain important even when a bone mass measurement is available. A previous fracture is an important predictor of further fracture, irrespective of BMD. Similarly, a family history of hip fracture (i.e. sibling or maternal hip fracture) is strongly associated with fracture risk. The SOFt study has also shown that current smoking status and inability to rise from a chair unaided are significant fracture risk factors.

For women between 50 and 60 years two studies, one in Scotland and the other in Finland, have confirmed the importance of a prior fracture as being an indicator of increased risk, as well as low bone mass.[40,41] Further, among these women an early or surgical menopause was noted as being an important fracture risk factor.

A risk factor that is particularly important both economically and clinically is the diagnosis of an incident vertebral fracture. Patients with a confirmed vertebral fracture have an extremely high risk of further fracture. Indeed, such patients have about a 20% absolute risk of sustaining another vertebral fracture within 12 months. As well as an elevated risk of subsequent vertebral fractures these patients are also at much greater risk of hip and other nonvertebral fractures. Because they have such a high fracture risk, treatment with most effective therapies is almost always bound to be cost-effective. Indeed, treatment may even be cost-saving, that is the costs of treatment are outweighed by the subsequent savings due to avoiding the treatment costs of further fractures.

As well as individual clinical indicators of risk there are certain sections of the population that have an elevated fracture risk above that of the general population. People in residential accommodation have an elevated risk of fracture as do patients taking oral steroid therapy. Thus, for example, a patient who has low bone mass and is taking oral steroids is almost certainly at greater fracture risk compared with the patient who has low bone mass alone.

Clinical risk factors are important economically because they present a simple and inexpensive method of targeting both BMD diagnostic methods and treatments. Some treatments such as estrogens can be cost-effectively targeted simply on the basis of risk factors, such as an early menopause, whilst others, namely the bisphosphonates probably almost always require a BMD measurement before a treatment decision is made efficiently.

CONCLUSIONS

Until relatively recently, hormone replacement therapy (HRT) was seen as the main method of treating and preventing osteoporotic fractures. Whilst recent data have now confirmed that HRT does, indeed, reduce the incidence of fractures, the expected benefit of hormones on cardiovascular endpoints has not materialized. This makes HRT a relatively non cost-effective therapy for a population approach of fracture prevention. However, the absolute harm of HRT in terms of adverse events, such as breast cancer and cardiovascular disease, is low, therefore among women at high risk of fracture where the absolute benefit of fracture prevention is high, and given that HRT is relatively inexpensive it may still be a cost-effective treatment.

The class of therapies that have the greatest amount of clinical and economic evidence to support their use are the bisphosphonates. The economic evidence suggests that for patients with established osteoporosis (i.e low BMD and existing fragility fractures) their use may not only be effective but, in some circumstances, can actually reduce health care costs. Given that the comparison treatment in many of the bisphosphonate trials was actually calcium and vitamin D supplementation this would make the bisphosphonates more cost-effective than calcium and vitamin D supplementation alone in women at high risk of fracture.

On the other hand, calcium and vitamin D supplementation is relatively inexpensive and therefore would seem to be a relatively cost-effective treatment for people who have an elevated non-BMD risk of fracture. For instance, people resident in sheltered accommodation may, cost-effectively, benefit from such supplements.

REFERENCES

1. Ades AE, Sculpher M, Gibb DM, Ratcliffe GJ. Cost effectiveness analysis of antenatal HIV screening in the United Kingdom. *BMJ* 1999;**319**: 1230–4.

2. Drummond MF, Torrance GW, Stoddart GL. *Methods for the Economic Evaluation of Health Care Programmes.* Oxford University Press, 1995.

3. Meltzer D. Accounting for future costs in medical cost-effectiveness analysis. *J Health Econ* 1997;**16**:33–64.

4. Gold MR, Siegel JE, Russell LB, Weinstein MC. Cost-effectiveness in health and medicine. Oxford University Press, 1996.

5. Robinson R. Cost-benefit analysis. *BMJ* 1993;**307**:924–6.

6. Briggs A, Sculpher M, Buxton M. Uncertainty in the economic evaluation of health care technologies: the role of sensitivity analysis. *Health Econ* 1994;**3**:95–104.

7. Briggs A, Gray AM. Handling uncertainty. *Health Technol Assess* 1999;3(2): 1–134.

8. Briggs AH. Handling uncertainty in cost-effectiveness models. *Pharmacoeconomics* 2000;**17**:479–500.

9. Van Hout BA, Al MJ, Gordon GS, Rutten FFH. Costs, effects and C/E ratios alongside a clinical trial. *Health Econ* 1994;**3**:309–19.

10. Fenwick E, Claxton K, Sculpher M. Representing uncertainty: the role of cost-effectiveness acceptability curves. *Health Econ* 2000;**10**:779–87.

11. Iglesias CP, Torgerson DJ, Bearne A, Bose U. The cost utility of bisphosphonate treatment in established osteoporosis *QJM* 2002;**95**: 305–11.

12. Fleurence R, Torgerson DJ, Reid DM. Cost-effectiveness of hormone replacement therapy for fracture prevention in young postmenopausal women: an economic analysis based on a prospective cohort study. *Osteoporos Int* 2002;**13**:637–43.

13. Torgerson DJ, Bell-Syer SEM. Hormone replacement therapy and prevention of nonvertebral fractures: A meta-analysis of randomized trials. *JAMA* 2001;**285**:289–97.

14. Torgerson DJ, Bell-Syer SEM. Hormone replacement therapy and prevention of vertebral fractures: a meta-analysis of randomised trials. *BMC Musculoskeletal Dis* 2001;**2**:7.

15. Torgerson DJ, Bell-Syer SEM, Porthouse J. Hormone replacement therapy and prevention of fractures: is age of starting therapy important? In:

Schnieder HPG, ed. *Menopause: State of the Art.* 108–14.

16. Rossouw JE, Anderson GL, Prentice RL et al. Risks and benefits of estrogen plus progestin in healthy post-menopausal women: principal results from the Women's Health Initiative randomized controlled trial. *JAMA* 2002;**288**:321–33.

17. Torgerson DJ, Reid DM. The economics of osteoporosis and its treatment. *Pharmacoeconomics* 1997;**11**:126–38.

18. Hulley S, Grady D, Bush T et al. Randomised trial of estrogen and progestin for secondary prevention of coronary heart disease in post-menopausal women. *JAMA* 1998;**280**:605–13.

19. Torgerson DJ, Iglesias CP, Reid DM. The economics of fracture prevention. In: Barlow DH, Francis RM, Miles A, eds. *The Effective Management of Osteoporosis.* London: Aesculapius Medical Press, 2001.

20. The Women's Health Initiative Steering Committee. Effects of conjugated equine estrogens in postmenopausal women with hysterectomy. *JAMA* 2004;**291**:1701–12.

21. McClung MR, Geusens P, Miller PD et al. Effect of risedronate on the risk of hip fracture in elderly women. *N Engl J Med* 2001;**344**:333–40.

22. Black DM, Cummings SR, Karpf DB et al. Randomised trial of effect of alendronate on risk of fracture in women with existing vertebral fractures. *Lancet* 1996;**348**:1535–41.

23. Cummings SR, Black DM, Thompson DE et al. Effect of alendronate on risk of fracture in women with low bone density but without fractures. *JAMA* 1998;**280**:2077–82.

24. Cranney A, Guyatt G, Krolicki N et al. A meta-analysis of etidronate for the treatment of postmenopausal osteoporosis. *Osteoporos Int* 2001;**12**:140–51.

25. Ankjaer-Jensen A, Johnell O. Prevention of osteoporosis: cost-effectiveness of different pharmaceutical treatments. *Osteoporos Int* 1996;**6**:265–75.

26. Francis RM, Anderson FH, Torgerson DJ. A comparison of the effectiveness and cost of treatment for vertebral fractures in women. *Br J Rheumatol* 1995;**34**(12):1167–71.

27. Rodriguez EC, Fidalgo Garcia ML, Rubio CS. [A cost-effectiveness analysis of alendronate compared to placebo in the prevention of hip fracture] (in Spanish). *Aten Primaria* 1999;**24**:390–6.

28. Visentin P, Ciravegna R, Fabris F. Estimating the cost per avoided hip fracture by osteoporosis treatment in Italy. *Maturitas* 1997;**26**(3):185–92.

29. Chapuy MC, Arlot ME, Duboeuf F et al. Vitamin D3 and calcium to prevent hip fractures in the elderly women. *N Engl J Med* 1992;**327**:1637–42.

30. Dawson-Hughes B, Harris SS, Krall EA, Dallal GE. Effect of calcium and vitamin D supplementation on bone density in men and women 65 years of age or older. *N Engl J Med* 1997;**337**:670–6.

31. Heikinheimo RJ, Inkovaara JA, Harju EJ et al. Annual injection of vitamin D and fractures of aged bones. *Calcif Tissue Int* 1992;**51**:105–10.

32. Lips P, Graafmans WC, Ooms ME, Bezemer PD, Bouter LM. Vitamin D supplementation and fracture incidence in elderly persons. A randomized, placebo-controlled clinical trial. *Ann Intern Med* 1996;**124**:400–6.

33. Geelhoed E, Harris A, Prince R. Cost-effectiveness analysis of hormone replacement therapy and lifestyle intervention for hip fracture. *Aust J Public Health* 1994;**18**:153–60.

34. Torgerson DJ, Kanis JA. Cost-effectiveness of preventing hip fractures in the elderly population using vitamin D and calcium. *QJM* 1995;**88**:135–9.

35. Bendich A, Leader S, Muhuri P. Supplemental calcium for the prevention of hip fracture: potential health economic benefits. *Clin Ther* 1999;**21**:1058–72.

36. Torgerson DJ, Donaldson C, Reid DM. Using economics to prioritize research: a case study of randomized trials for the prevention of hip

fractures due to osteoporosis. *J Health Serv Res Policy* 1996;**1**:141–6.

37. Geelhoed E, Harris A, Prince R. Cost-effectiveness analysis of hormone replacement therapy and lifestyle intervention for hip fracture. *Aust J Pub Health* 1994;**18**:153–60.

38. Trivedi, DP, Doll R, Khaw KT. Effect of four monthly oral vitamin D (cholecalciferol) supplementation on fractures and mortality in men and women living in the community: randomised double blind controlled trial. *BMJ* 2003;**326**:46.

39. Eddy DM, Johnston CC, Cummings SR et al. Osteoporosis: cost-effectiveness analysis and review of the evidence for prevention, diagnosis and treatment. *Osteoporos Int* 1998; (Suppl 4): S1–S88.

40. Torgerson DJ, Campbell MK, Thomas RE, Reid DM. Prediction of perimenopausal fractures by bone mineral density and other risk factors. *J Bone Miner Res* 1996;**11**:293–7.

41. Kroger H, Huopio J, Honkanen R et al. Prediction of fracture risk using axial bone mineral density in a perimenopausal population: a prospective study. *J Bone Miner Res* 1995;**10**:302–6.

7
Strategies for prevention

Stephen Gehlbach

The development of strategies to prevent fragility fractures requires not only identifying risk factors responsible but documenting that proposed interventions can lower risk and improve outcomes. Both these domains have generated large amounts of complex, sometimes inconsistent literature. As indicated in previous chapters, a variety of individual risk factors has been associated with increased fracture risk. Principal among these, and the focus of much of the work on osteoporosis, is bone mineral density (BMD). The risk of fracture clearly increases as BMD declines. However, many clinical factors relating to fracture risk also contribute, including physical characteristics, such as age and weight, features of history like maternal or personal history of fracture, and such habits as exercise and smoking. As risk factors are multiple, so are possible approaches for reducing risk. These range from the pharmacologic interventions outlined in Chapter 5 to attempts to modify diet and habits to programs to reduce the incidence of falls.

Several national and international organizations have taken on the challenge of sorting through the substantial body of accumulated information to propose recommendations to guide clinical practice. Four that offer credibility as well as geographic diversity are: The National Osteoporosis Foundation of the United States (NOF),[1] the Osteoporosis Society of Canada (OSC),[2] the Royal College of Physicians of Great Britain (RCP)[3] and the European Foundation for Osteoporosis and Bone Disease (EFFO).[4] These groups have conducted extensive reviews, evaluated the literature and published recommendations. Guidelines are based on the importance of the risks identified and the effectiveness of the potential interventions.

RISK FACTORS

The expert panels have considered both behavioral or environmental risks that are potentially subject to modification and intrinsic risks that may be attenuated by pharmacologic therapy.

Five factors related to behaviors or environment have been extensively evaluated for their relationship to fragility fractures: nutrition, physical activity, cigarette smoking, alcohol consumption, and falls. Several published literature reviews and meta-analyses have served to guide recommendations.

Nutrition

A 1997 meta-analysis reviewed 23 observational studies that related dietary calcium to fracture outcomes (18 studies were of hip fracture and 5 of other fracture sites).[5] Individual study findings varied somewhat, but the five population-based cohort studies of hip fracture, as well as the overall pooled risk estimate, showed declining fracture risk with increasing dietary calcium. The pooled odds ratio indicated a 4% reduction in hip fracture risk for each 300 mg increase in daily dietary calcium intake. This value is equivalent to one glass of milk per day. The benefit from calcium is reinforced by results of several small clinical trials with calcium supplements which show reduced fractures among those receiving supplements.[5]

Adequate intake of calcium as well as sufficient amounts of vitamin D are related to bone health and the risk of fragility fractures. Providing appropriate levels of these two nutrients either in the diet or as supplements appears to lessen fracture risk. For both men and women over 50 years of age a total intake of 1200–1500 mg of calcium and 400–800 IU of vitamin D (preferably in the D_3 form) is generally recommended. Given the less than optimal dietary intake for most middle-aged and older adults in Europe and North America this recommendation suggests the use of supplements. These are relatively low in cost and their use in individual patients, particularly those at increased fracture risk seems reasonable.

Physical activity

Physical activity appears to protect again fracture, particularly at the hip. A systematic review of 14 case control and 4 follow-up studies[6] found a consistently lower risk of fracture among those engaged in greater amounts of leisure time activity. However, the interrelationships of activity with other risks such as weight, and smoking make assessment of its independent role difficult. Those who are active differ in many respects from the sedentary, and so, although many of the studies adjusted results for known associated risks, residual confounding is possible. Benefits of exercise appear related to the positive effects of weight bearing on bone density and quality, and there are indications that only activities that place substantial stress on bones succeed in maintaining or enhancing bone density. Some benefit from exercise is certainly gained from a reduced risk of falls that comes with improved muscle strength, balance and co-ordination.

Programs that aim to lower fracture risks through exercise have been challenging to evaluate. Reported studies are hampered by small sample sizes and large attrition rates. The data point to benefits for BMD at both the spine and hip.[6] However, as this effect appears most strongly when exercise places stress on the bone (impact vs non-impact activities), the value of much adult exercise (swimming, cycling, yoga) to enhancing bone strength remains open to question. Still, as even non-impact exercise may improve strength and balance and lead to lower rates of falls, potential benefits extend beyond direct effects on bone. Given the additional, accepted value of exercise on the cardiovascular system, patients should be encouraged to engage in activities that will increase exercise and have a reasonable likelihood of being continued.

Cigarette smoking and alcohol use

A 1997 meta-analysis reviewed 29 cross-sectional studies that related smoking to bone density and 19 cohort and case control efforts that reported comparative risks of hip fracture in smokers and non-smokers.[7] The authors found a modest annual increase in bone loss among postmenopausal women who smoked compared with non-smokers (no such effect was observed in premenopausal women). The effect was cumulative with a 2% decline in bone density for every 10 year increment of increasing age. Current smokers showed an excess risk of hip fracture from age 50 years that rose to 17% at age 65 years to 41% at age 70 years, 71% at age 80 years and was 2-fold for women reaching 90 years of age. Although cigarette smoking is less prevalent at older ages, it is estimated to be responsible for 13%, or 1 in 8, of fractures.[7] Data on smoking and fracture risk in men are less robust but suggest a pattern similar to that in women. The mechanism by which smoking influences risk is uncertain, but findings of the meta-analysis persist when possible confounding factors, known to be related to smoking, such as lower weight, anti-estrogen effects and physical activity were considered.

The heavy use of alcohol has been associated with increased fracture risk.[8,9] As alcohol intake is closely associated with smoking, poor diet, and propensity to fall, it has been difficult to identify its independent influence on fracture. Inconsistent findings from several studies have shown both slightly increased fracture risk and a protective effect from low and moderate alcohol consumption.[9] Evidence of higher risk among heavy drinkers is more consistent but difficult to evaluate due to the complex interrelationship of the factors mentioned above, particularly the increased propensity to fall.

The data that relate smoking to fracture risk suggest the usual solution. Though generally rates of cigarette smoking decline with age and older women in particular have low prevalence, the risk of fracture adds yet another to the list of adverse health effects of smoking and provides another reason for the physician to encourage cessation. The data for alcohol are less compelling and a moderate intake does not appear to increase fracture risk. Heavy drinking is a problem that, like smoking, should be curtailed for a variety of reasons.

Falls

Although fragility fractures are defined as due to minimal trauma, some stress upon a fragile bone is generally required to precipitate a fracture. In many cases, particularly with hip and wrist fractures, fall from a standing height is involved. Such falls become more common as people age. As many as 30% of people 65 years and older experience a fall each year.[10] Although less than 10% of these falls result in fracture, the cumulative total is substantial. The likelihood of falling increases as individuals age, experience declining health and impaired vision, and lose muscle strength and balance. Side effects from medications, such as orthostatic hypotension, sedation, or disequilibrium contribute to falls.[11] The outcome of any fall depends upon its type and direction and the impact that results. Padding, either natural (adipose tissue) or artificial (hip protectors) that diffuses force reduces the likelihood of fracture.

Programs aimed at reducing falls have taken the form of exercise and balance activities as well as interventions intended to reduce environmental hazards, such as inadequate lighting, slippery surfaces, and loose carpeting. Adjustment of medications and use of hip protectors to reduce impact on the bones of those who do fall have also been evaluated. Although results from individual studies have been mixed, several reviews indicate that approaches that increase muscle strength and balance, reduce the use of psychotropic medications and remediate household environmental hazards have had success.[11] Use of hip protectors in residential settings reduces the likelihood of fractures amongst those who fall but compliance is difficult to maintain.[12]

Intrinsic risks and pharmacologic intervention

Identifying patients who have a risk profile that will benefit from pharmacologic intervention is the practitioner's greatest challenge. When to obtain bone density determinations, how to incorporate clinical factors in risk determination and management decisions, and when to initiate pharmacologic intervention are questions at the heart of the issue.

Bone mineral density determinations and clinical risk factors

BMD is now the focal point for most strategies to reduce fragility fractures. The expert groups rely heavily on BMD results to make their treatment recommendations. Intrinsic patient characteristics including a variety of disease and disability states and certain medications, as well as some of the behavioral factors noted above are used to determine which patients are best candidates for BMD examination. The factors deemed to carry significant risk for osteoporosis can be seen in Table 7.1.

The National Osteoporosis Foundation (NOF) suggests that BMD be obtained for all postmenopausal women 65 years and older, as well as 'younger

Table 7.1   Expert group identification of risk factors for osteoporosis

Risk factor	Endorsing organization			
	NOF	OSC	RCP	EFFO
Age	M	M	x	x
Personal history of fragility fracture	M	M	x	x
Fragility fracture in 1st degree relative	M	M	x	x
Low body weight/body mass index	M	a	x	x
Current smoking	M	a	x	x
Chronic corticosteroid therapy	M	M	x	x
Impaired vision	a			
Early menopause (<45 years)	a	M	x	x
Dementia	a			
Poor health/frailty	a			
Recent falls	a	M		
Low calcium intake	a	a		x
Low physical activity	a			
Excessive alcohol consumption	a		a	x
Malabsorption syndrome	M			
Primary hyperparathyroidism	M			
Radiographic evidence of osteopenia	M		x	x
Hypogonadism	M		x	x
Rheumatoid arthritis		a		
Past hyperthyroidism		a		
Chronic anticonvulsant therapy		a		
Weight loss > 10% of weight at age 25		a		
Chronic heparin therapy		a		
Excessive caffeine intake		a		
Loss of height			x	x
Prolonged amenorrhea			x	x
Chronic disorders associated with osteoporosis	a		x	x

x = ungraded risk factor
M = major risk factor
a = additional or secondary risk factor

NOF = National (US) Osteoporosis Foundation
OSC = Osteoporosis Society of Canada
RCP = Royal College of Physicians
EFFO = European Foundation for Osteoporosis and Bone Disease

postmenopausal women who have one or more risk factors,' as well as for those who have 'suffered a fragility fracture.'[1] The risk factors fall into 'major' and 'additional' categories. Major risks include, 'personal history of fracture as an adult, history of fragility fracture in a first degree relative, low body weight (less than 127 lbs [58 kg]), current smoking and use of oral corticosteroid therapy for more than 3 months.' These are strongly supported by research evidence and generally add independently to the risk of fracture. 'Additional' risk factors, however, such as impaired vision, estrogen deficiency at an early age and dementia, are less well established as independent risks.

The Osteoporosis Society of Canada (OSC) identifies four 'key' factors – age, low bone mineral density, prior fragility fracture, and family history of osteoporosis that 'stand out as predictors of fracture related to osteoporosis.'[2] It also recognizes the risk of glucocorticoid therapy. The Canadian group suggests BMD testing over the age of 65 years and for those (including men) over 50 years who have at least one major or two minor risk factors. Their list consists of 10 major factors (including age greater than 65 years), and 10 minor ones. Agreements with the NOF list are evident, as are the differences. Among major risk factors considered major by the Canadians but not the Americans, for example, are medical conditions, such as hypogonadism, malabsorption syndrome, and primary hyperparathyroidism. Listed with the minor risks are smoking and low body weight, factors that the NOF considers strong independent predictors of fracture risk.

The Royal College of Physicians (RCP) notes that 'at present there is no universally accepted policy for screening to identify patients with osteoporosis.'[3] Its experts recommend a 'case finding strategy' in which patients are identified 'because of a fragility fracture or by the presence of strong risk factors.' Included in their risk factor list are 12 items; most, but not all, of which overlap with NOF and OSC items (see Table 7.1). The RCP, however, stops short of recommending BMD testing to any group on the basis of age alone.

The Report on Osteoporosis in the European Community[4] agrees with the RCP. It argues that 'population-based screening for osteoporosis cannot at present be justified in any age group,' and, 'In clinical practice a higher risk strategy is thus adopted to select individuals for bone densitometry, based on the presence of strong clinical and historical risk factors.'[4] These factors are also seen in Table 7.1.

Pharmacologic intervention

Recommendations on when to provide drug treatment to prevent fragility fractures are largely predicated on results obtained from BMD testing. The NOF recommends 'initiating therapy to lessen fracture risk in postmenopausal women with central dual-energy X-ray absorptiometry (DXA) T-scores below -2.0 in the absence of risk factors and in women with T-scores below -1.5 if one or more risk factors is present.' They also suggest 'considering postmenopausal women with prior vertebral or hip fractures as candidates for treatment.'[1] Their 'action range' for BMD, which extends into the 'osteopenic' designation, is broader than is suggested by other expert groups. The RCP suggests intervening 'within the range for osteoporosis (T-score less than -2.5).'[3] The Osteoporosis Society of Canada identifies bisphosphonates, hormone replacement therapy, and raloxifene as effective agents at reducing bone loss and preventing osteoporotic fractures in postmenopausal women and in osteoporotic men but defers with respect to just which patients should be offered treatment.[2]

BONE MINERAL DENSITY AND RISK

These recommendations illustrate several of the limitations encountered in developing strategic approaches to identifying and managing patients with increased fracture risk. The first is the reliance on BMD as chief arbiter of risk. Current guidelines lean heavily on BMD to guide pharmacologic treatment, albeit thresholds of intervention vary. The trend is to consider those with BMDs with T-scores of −2.5 or less as candidates for treatment, though the NOF is more aggressive with a threshold T-score of −2.0. Some latitude is given when previous fractures or 'other risk factors', such as chronic glucocorticoid use, are present. The problem becomes that BMD cut points of −2.5 or even −2.0 fail to identify many patients who will experience fractures. Data from the large, cohort Study of Osteoporotic Fractures (SOF) demonstrate that over 30% of fractures occur in women with density scores above the NOF threshold of −2.0.[13]

The SOF enrolled almost 10,000 white women aged 65 years and over, identified from population-based listings for geographic disparate locations in the USA during 1986–88. These women were assessed at entry and followed at 4 monthly intervals for occurrence of fragility fractures. Among almost 8000 of these women for whom femoral BMD measures were available, there were 231 hip fractures during 5 years. Only 46% of these were in women with BMDs in the 'osteoporotic' range.[13] A subsequent report by the SOF group[14] substantiates that for a variety of skeletal sites the proportion of fractures that can be attributed to osteoporosis (a BMD T-score of <2.5) is low, ranging from less than 10% to 44%. Clearly other factors (included in the list in Table 7.1) exert a role in fracture risk.

COMBINING RISK FACTORS

Almost 30 individual characteristics linked to fractures have been identified by expert groups. These factors are often interrelated, however, so that when more than one is present, the independent role of each may not be clear. Moreover, risks co-exist in differing combinations among different patients. Thus a second problem highlighted by current guidelines, and major challenge to developing prevention strategies, lies in integrating the many variations into a composite risk. A number of investigators have employed multi-variable statistical techniques to build scoring systems that assess the influence of each risk factor while controlling or adjusting for the presence of the others. Factors that are found to contribute independently to risk are weighted by importance (as determined in the modeling) and allocated points. Each patient is then evaluated and receives a score, based on accumulated points, that predicts the risk of fracture.

Some scoring systems have been designed to predict low BMD (osteoporosis, as defined by the WHO) in the expectation that these scores will assist clinicians in identifying patients who will benefit from bone density referrals to confirm suspected diagnoses.[15,16] Other researchers have targeted fractures as the outcome of importance.[13,17] In these schemes BMD becomes one of the predictor variables. The latter approach has the dual virtues of utilizing easily obtained 'clinical variables,' such as age, sex and weight, and personal history to estimate risk before resorting to the added expense of a bone density determination, as well as predicting the outcome (fracture) of clinical importance.

Table 7.2 Multi-variable hip fracture predictors[17]

Predictor	Beta	Odds ratio (95% CI)	Points
Model including bone mineral density			
Intercept	–	–	–
Age (5 years)[a]	10.20	1.8 (1.5–2.3)	6
Gender (female)	0.61	2.6 (1.0–6.4)	9
Height (5 cm class)[b]	0.94	1.5 (1.1–1.9)	4
Use of a walking aid (yes/no)	0.39	2.7 (1.4–5.2)	10
Current cigarette smoking (yes/no)	0.98	2.2 (1.1–4.4)	8
Bone mineral density (0.05 g/cm^2)[d]	0.80	1.5 (1.3–1.7)	4
	0.39		
Model excluding bone mineral density			
Intercept	−9.60	–	5
Age (5 years)[a]	0.70	2.0 (1.6–2.5)	7
Sex (female)	1.20	3.3 (1.3–8.3)	12
Height (5 cm)[b]	0.40	1.5 (1.1–2.0)	4
Weight (5 kg)[c]	0.17	1.2 (1.0–1.4)	2
Use of a walking aid (yes/no)	1.08	2.9 (1.5–5.8)	11
Current cigarette smoking (yes/no)	0.87	2.4 (1.2–4.6)	9

[a]Age classes 0 to 6 are <60–64, etc, to ≥85 years
[b]Height classes 0 to 5 are <1.60–1.64 etc., to ≥1.80 m.
[c]Weight classes 0 to 9 are ≥95, 90–94, etc., to <55 kg
[d]Bone mineral density classes 0 to 9 are ≥1.00, 0.95–0.99, etc 55 kg, to <0.60 g/cm^2.

Box 7.1 Example of risk score calculation

A 60-year-old women with a height of 1.72 m, who walks without aid, does not smoke, and has a bone density of 0.68 g/cm^2 will have a risk score of
$$1 \times 6 + 9 + 3 \times 4 + 7 \times 4 = 55.$$

Two large population-based studies, one in Europe and one in North America, provide useful illustrations of how variables can be combined to estimate fracture risk. A cohort of over 5000 women and men aged 55 years and above from a Netherlands community was extensively evaluated from 1990 through 1993, then followed over a 4 year period for the occurrence of hip fracture.[17] Ten factors assessed at entry were associated with the outcome. After these were modeled in multi-variable equations, the factors seen in Table 7.2 emerged as independent contributors to fracture risk. Age, sex, height, use of an aid for walking, and current cigarette smoking are included as are nine categories of bone density. As seen in the table, the rounded estimates of the beta coefficients (weights of the factors) when multiplied by 10 become 'points' given to each factor. Points in turn are multiplied by the category value and summed to make a composite score (see Box 7.1). Within the Dutch population on which the scoring system was devised, subjects' scores range from 6 to 103 with a median value of 43. The scheme performs well in discriminating patients who are at high and low risk of fracture. Those with a score of less than 50, for example, have a chance of only 1 in 1000 of sustaining a hip fracture over a 4 year interval. This risk increases 100-fold for those with scores of 75 or higher; their risk of hip fracture is 10% as Figure 7.1 demonstrates.

In developing their prediction scheme the investigators also created a set of scores that excluded BMD. Values for this model are also shown in Table 7.2 and Figure 7.1. When BMD is excluded, model variables remain the same with the addition of weight as an independent contributor. Performance of the two models is similar as Figure 7.1 illustrates.

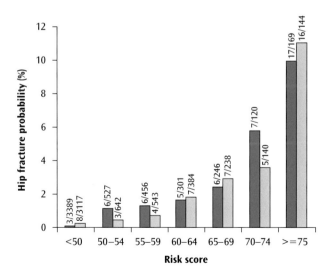

Figure 7.1

Four year probability of hip fracture by category of risk score. Solid bars represent score including bone mineral density (BMD) determination; shaded bars represent score without BMD determination. (Data from Burger et al, 1999.[17])

Data from the sub-set of US-based SOF subjects with hip DXA measurements available were also used to produce multi-variable derived prediction models.[13] Twenty potential risk factors were included in the modeling. Their results compiled into the 'FRACTURE Index' are shown in Table 7.3. Like the Dutch models, age, weight and cigarette smoking appeared as independent risks, as did an indicator of physical condition, in this instance 'using arms to stand from a chair' instead of 'using a walking aid.' Significant additions to the

Table 7.3 FRACTURE Index questions and scoring[13]	
	Point value
1. What is your current age?	
Less than 65	0
65–69	1
70–74	2
75–79	3
80–84	4
85 or older	5
2. Have you broken any bones after age 50?	
Yes	1
No/Don't know	0
3. Has your mother had a hip fracture after age 50?	
Yes	1
No/Don't know	0
4. Do you weigh 125 pounds or less?	
Yes	1
No	0
5. Are you currently a smoker?	
Yes	1
No	0
6. Do you usually need to use your arms to assist yourself in standing up from a chair?	
Yes	2
No/Don't know	0
If you have a current bone density (BMD) assessment, then answer the next question.	
7. BMD results: Total hip T-score	
T-score ≥ −1	0
T-score between −1 and −2	2
T-score between −2 and −2.5	3
T-score <22.5	4

SOF models are the history of maternal hip fracture after the age of 50 years and the personal history of a fracture in adult life.

As in the Dutch study, the American group built models that included and excluded BMD determinations. Scores from both FRACTURE Index models show good discrimination for fracture risk as Figure 7.2 displays. Subjects with scores in the lowest quintile have a 5 year risk of hip fracture of about 0.5% compared with a 14-fold increased risk of 8.5% for scores in the highest quintile. Good separation for those at high and low risk of vertebral fracture was also demonstrated. As with the Dutch models, adding BMD values to the models derived from clinical variables alone improves performance, although not dramatically.

A particular strength of the SOF study is the validation of the instrument in a different population. The scoring system was applied to 6600 women aged 75 years and older from five regions in France who were participants in a hip fracture follow-up study.[13] Although this group was on average 10 years older than SOF participants, the models, both with and without BMD, showed good discrimination with 23-fold and 6-fold increases in estimated risk, respectively between lowest and highest quintiles.

Other efforts to combine risk factors have found more than 20 characteristics that predict increased fracture risk in multivariate models.[18–21] In addition

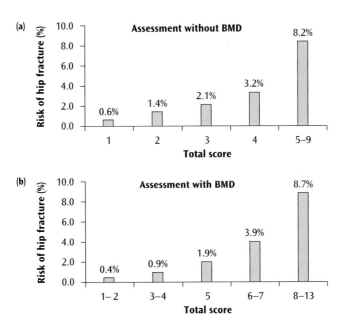

Figure 7.2

Five-year risk of hip fracture by quintiles of FRACTURE Index risk score without (a), and with (b) addition of bone mineral density (BMD) determination.

to those observed by Black et al[13] and Burger et al,[17] activities of daily living (ADLs), cognition, propensity to fall, poor overall health status, history of stroke, seizure disorder, and several different medications have been identified. In four of five of these investigations simple counts of increasing number of risk factors have been shown to demonstrate increasing risk. In data from the Duke Established Population for Epidemiologic Studies of the Elderly in the USA the presence of one of nine factors carries a fracture risk of 1.8 while four factors increase risk to almost 10.[18] Findings from the General Practice Research Database in the UK indicate that the presence of three or more of 11 medical risk factors (made up of diagnoses and medications) raises the risk of vertebral fracture 8-fold and of hip fracture by a factor of 4.6 when compared to patients with none of the attributes.[19] Neither of the latter studies included measurements of BMD.

Models that avoid reliance on BMD appear promising. However, the prospect that preventive treatment decisions might be made without obtaining BMD determinations is mitigated by concern that anti-resorptive agents may not be equally effective across a range of BMD. Data from randomized trials of alendronate[22] and risedronate[23] suggest that the bisphosphonates have little effect on fracture reduction among subjects with BMD levels above the osteoporotic range.

RELATIVE RISK, ABSOLUTE RISK AND RISK DIFFERENCE

Identifying patients at increased likelihood of fracture is commonly expressed in terms of relative risk: the ratio of occurrence of fracture among those with the factor or characteristic over the occurrence in those without the characteristic. Relative risk (also referred to as risk ratio) estimates the potency or strength of an association between a factor and an outcome. A BMD in the osteoporotic range carries a risk ratio of 9.6 for hip fracture compared with a relative risk of 1.7 for cigarette smoking, for example, suggesting that low BMD has the greater impact on producing fracture risk.

However, relative risk alone does not provide sufficient information for informed clinical decisions. It fails to convey an important dimension of risk, the absolute value. What is the actual magnitude of risk, the frequency with which the outcome or disease occurs? Table 7.4 shows data on the 10 year fracture rates for women who are 50 years old and women aged 70 years by two levels of BMD, 'osteoporotic' and 'normal'. The relative risks for the two groups are similar (3.7 and 4.2 respectively), but the absolute rates of fracture appear quite different. The 10 year risk of fracture is 2-fold higher for older osteoporotic women. This has important implications for any preventive strategy. If an intervention were able to reduce the 'osteoporotic' risk to the 'normal' level, more fractures would be averted in the older women (22.7 per 100 compared with 10.1 per 100). This *risk difference* can be expressed in the useful notation 'number needed to treat' (NNT) to avoid one fracture (the

Table 7.4   Ten year risk of fracture associated with osteoporosis for 50- and 70-year-old women[24]

	50 years old	70 years old
Absolute risk (per 100)		
Osteoporosis (BMD, T-score<−2.5 SD)	13.9	29.8
Normal (BMD, T-score=mean*)	3.8	7.1
Relative risk	3.7	4.2
Risk difference (per 100)	10.1	22.7
NNT	9.9	4.4

*mean BMD for young adult
BMD, bone mineral density; SD, standard deviation; NNT, number needed to treat to prevent one fracture (1/risk difference).

reciprocal of the risk difference). Ten younger women would require treatment to avert one fracture compared with four in the older age group.

Recent thinking has moved away from describing fracture risk in relative terms.[25] A more informative approach is to estimate the likelihood that an individual with a given constellation of factors (age, BMD, prior fracture) will sustain a fracture over a particular period of time. This means constructing an estimate of absolute risk and utilizing risk differences as a basis for evaluating intervention strategies. The principal value to employing absolute risk is its transparent role in economic analyses. As noted in Chapter 6, the cost-effectiveness and cost-utility calculations that are assuming essential roles in

Table 7.5   Estimated 10 year risk of fracture at various ages in the UK[26]

	Age (years)	Fracture risk (%)			
		Any fracture	Radius/ulna	Hip/femur	Vertebral
Women					
	50	9.8	3.2	0.3	0.3
	60	13.3	4.9	1.1	0.6
	70	17.0	5.6	3.4	1.3
	80	21.7	5.5	8.7	1.6
Men					
	50	7.1	1.1	0.2	0.2
	60	5.7	0.9	0.4	0.3
	70	6.2	0.9	1.4	0.5
	80	8.0	0.9	2.9	0.7

both clinical and policy decision-making depend upon the values obtained from comparisons of the risk differences of alternative interventions. The time interval over which risk is determined is arbitrary, but 10 years has been proposed as a practical length of time in which to observe maximum benefits of a treatment program.[25] Couching estimates in longer frames, such as lifetime risk presume extended benefits that are not yet demonstrated and ignore the improvements in treatment approaches that seem likely in coming years. Table 7.5 gives an example of 10 year fracture risk estimates that provides a useful baseline of absolute risk from which intervention strategies could be formulated.

CONCLUSIONS

Where does all this leave the clinician? Well-researched guidelines are available that offer prevention strategies that are based on summaries of present knowledge. However, the ongoing stream of new research findings make continuing updating of any such guidelines essential. Moreover, some may find frustration at the lack of concordance among expert groups or wish for more direction in how to include and weight particular patient characteristics or utilize the presence of multiple risk factors effectively. On the other hand the non-prescriptive nature of the recommendations leaves flexibility for individual physician-patient decisions.

Several findings do emerge with ample clarity. There is reasonable concordance of opinion that individuals, both men and women, with BMD findings in the osteoporotic range (T-scores less than −2.5) are candidates for pharmacologic intervention. Because the agents outlined in Chapter 5 exert their influence largely by preventing bone resorption and maintaining or enhancing bone mass, this approach seems sound. It is on individuals with demonstrated low BMD that these agents appear to have most benefit. The increasing risk of fracture that comes with the 'clinical' features of being female and white, advancing age, having low body weight, a personal or maternal history of fragility fracture, or use of long-term glucocorticoids is also well established. The fact that these factors contribute independently and additively to fracture risk suggest that even simple, unweighted cumulative scoring schemes can be helpful.

The efficacy of initiating treatment in such individuals without the aid of BMD results has yet to be documented. Neither treatment nor preventive trials based on results of clinical scoring systems have been reported. Still, the greatly increased fracture risk in older individuals with multiple risks suggests that in locations where BMD testing is not readily accessible, treatment could reasonably proceed on the basis of high clinical risk alone. Older women with prior fragility fractures or those on long-term glucocorticoids are particularly strong candidates.

The development of strategies to reduce osteoporotic fractures is a work in progress. More needs to be known about the effect of pharmacologic interventions across a range of clinical risks and BMD values as well as the applicability of multi-risk evaluation schemes to differing populations. The value of utilizing absolute risk figures to plan strategies needs to be explored. However, it appears that we are moving in the right direction towards the creation, validation and promulgation of preventive strategies that have the potential to reduce the burden of osteoporotic fracture in future generations.

REFERENCES

1. National Osteoporosis Foundation. *Physician's Guide to Prevention and Treatment of Osteoporosis.* Washington, DC: National Osteoporosis Foundation, 1998.
2. Brown JP, Josse RG. 2002 clinical practice guidelines for the diagnosis and management of osteoporosis in Canada. *CMAJ* 2002;**167**(Suppl 10): S1–S34.
3. Royal College of Physicians of London. *Osteoporosis Clinical Guidelines for Prevention and Treatment.* London: Royal College of Physicians of London, 1999.
4. Kanis JA, Delmas P, Burckhardt P, Cooper C, Torgerson D. Guidelines for diagnosis and management of osteoporosis. The European Foundation for Osteoporosis and Bone Disease. *Osteoporos Int* 1997;**7**(4): 390–406.
5. Cumming RG, Nevitt MC. Calcium for prevention of osteoporotic fractures in postmenopausal women. *J Bone Miner Res* 1997;**12**(9):1321–9.
6. Joakimsen RM, Magnus JH, Fonnebo V. Physical activity and predisposition for hip fractures: a review. *Osteoporos Int* 1997;**7**(6):503–13.
7. Law MR, Hackshaw AK. A meta-analysis of cigarette smoking, bone mineral density and risk of hip fracture: recognition of a major effect. *BMJ* 1997;**315**:841–6.
8. Bikle DD, Genant HK, Cann C, Recker RR, Halloran BP, Strewler GJ. Bone disease in alcohol abuse. *Ann Intern Med* 1985;**103**(1):42–8.
9. Naves Diaz M, O'Neill TW, Silman AJ. The influence of alcohol consumption on the risk of vertebral deformity. European Vertebral Osteoporosis Study Group. *Osteoporos Int* 1997; **7**(1):65–71.
10. Gillespie LD, Gillespie WJ, Robertson MC, Lamb SE, Cumming RG, Rowe BH. Interventions for preventing falls in elderly people (Cochrane Review). In: *The Cochrane Library, Issue 1.* Chichester, UK: Wiley, 2004.
11. Tinetti ME. Clinical practice. Preventing falls in elderly persons. *N Engl J Med* 2003;**348**(1):42–9.
12. Feder G, Cryer C, Donovan S, Carter Y. Guidelines for the prevention of falls in people over 65. The Guidelines' Development Group. *BMJ* 2000;**321**:1007–11.
13. Black DM, Steinbuch M, Palermo L et al. An assessment tool for predicting fracture risk in postmenopausal women. *Osteoporos Int* 2001;**12**(7): 519–28.
14. Stone KL, Seeley DG, Lui LY et al. BMD at multiple sites and risk of fracture of multiple types: long-term results from the Study of Osteoporotic Fractures. *J Bone Miner Res* 2003; **18**(11):1947–54.
15. Cadarette SM, Jaglal SB, Murray TM, McIsaac WJ, Joseph L, Brown JP. Evaluation of decision rules for referring women for bone densitometry by dual-energy X-ray absorptiometry. *JAMA* 2001;**286**(1):57–63.
16. Geusens P, Hochberg MC, van der Voort DJ et al. Performance of risk indices for identifying low bone density in postmenopausal women. *Mayo Clin Proc* 2002;**77**(7):629–37.
17. Burger H, De Laet CE, Weel AE,

Hofman A, Pols HA. Added value of bone mineral density in hip fracture risk scores. *Bone* 1999;**25**(3):369–74.

18. Colon-Emeric CS, Pieper CF, Artz MB. Can historical and functional risk factors be used to predict fractures in community-dwelling older adults? Development and validation of a clinical tool. *Osteoporos Int* 2002;**13**(12): 955–61.

19. van Staa TP, Leufkens HG, Cooper C. Utility of medical and drug history in fracture risk prediction among men and women. *Bone* 2002;**31**(4): 508–14.

20. McGrother CW, Donaldson MM, Clayton D, Abrams KR, Clarke M. Evaluation of a hip fracture risk score for assessing elderly women: the Melton Osteoporotic Fracture (MOF) study. *Osteoporos Int* 2002;**13**(1): 89–96.

21. Walter LC, Lui LY, Eng C, Covinsky KE. Risk of hip fracture in disabled community-living older adults. *J Am Geriatr Soc* Jan 2003;**51**(1):50–5.

22. Cummings SR, Black DM, Thompson DE et al. Effect of alendronate on risk of fracture in women with low bone density but without vertebral fractures: results from the Fracture Intervention Trial. *JAMA* 1998; **280**(24):2077–82.

23. McClung MR, Geusens P, Miller PD et al. Effect of risedronate on the risk of hip fracture in elderly women. Hip Intervention Program Study Group. *N Engl J Med* 2001;**344**(5):333–40.

24. Kanis JA, Johnell O, Oden A, Dawson A, De Laet C, Jonsson B. Ten year probabilities of osteoporotic fractures according to BMD and diagnostic thresholds. *Osteoporos Int* 2001; **12**(12):989–95.

25. Kanis JA, Black D, Cooper C et al. A new approach to the development of assessment guidelines for osteoporosis. *Osteoporos Int* 2002;**13**(7): 527–36.

26. van Staa TP, Dennison EM, Leufkens HG, Cooper C. Epidemiology of fractures in England and Wales. *Bone* 2001;**29**(6):517–22.

Index

Page numbers in *italics* indicate figures or tables.

activities of daily living, impact of fractures 19–20, *20*
aging
  BMD changes 13–14, *14*, 27–8, *28*
  demographic change and 22, *22*
  falls risk 106
  fracture frequency and 16, *16*, 17
  fracture risk and *47*, 47–8, *48*
  historical perspectives 2
  osteoporosis frequency and 13–14, *14*, 44, *45*
Albright, F 1–2
alcohol use 105
alendronate
  cost effectiveness 88, 89, *91*, 97
  efficacy *62*, *63*, 64–5
  vs other agents 73
  vs other treatments 72
alfacalcidol 67
alkaline phosphatase 32, 38–9
androgens 38

back pain 19
bisphosphonates 61–6, 73
  antifracture efficacy *62*, *63*
  cost effectiveness 88–9, *90–1*, 100
  indications 71
  safety 64
BMD *see* bone mineral density
body weight, low 98
bone 29–36
  components 29, *29*, 30–6
  cortical 29
  mineralization 32
  non-collagen proteins 31
  trabecular (spongy) 29–30
  turnover markers 38–9, 72
bone cells 32–6
  biochemical measures of activity 38–9
  conversation between 35–6
bone Gla protein (osteocalcin) 38, 39
bone mass
  age-related loss 28, *28*
  determinants 33, 39

peak 27, *28*
bone matrix 30–1
bone mineral density (BMD) 3–6
  accuracy of measurements 45
  age-related changes 13–14, *14*, 27–8, *28*
  defining osteoporosis 3, *4*, *4*, 44
  effects of therapy 72
  fracture risk and 109
  fracture risk assessment *45*, 45–8, *47*, *48*
  fracture risk stratification 52
  indications for measurement 106–8
  interpretation 6
  intervention thresholds 43–4, 71, 108–9, 116
  measurement sites 6, 44
  measurement techniques 3–4, *5*
  risk scoring 110, *110*, 111, 112–13, *113*, 114
  treatment monitoring 72
bone morphogenetic proteins (BMPs) 32
bone multicellular (or remodelling) units (BMU or BRU) 34, *35*
bone remodelling cycle 34, 36, *36*
breast cancer 60, 61, 87

calcitonin 33, 38
  cost effectiveness 97
  therapy *62*, *63*, 66
calcitriol 67
calcium
  balance 36–8
  cost effectiveness 92–7, *93–6*, 98, 100
  dietary intake 68–9, 104
  supplements 58
Canadian Multicentre Osteoporosis Study 14, 15
carbonic anhydrase 33
cardiovascular disease 60, 86–7
case finding strategies 43–4, 108
  optimization 52
cholecalciferol 37
clodronate 65, *91*
cognitive function 61
collagen 29, 30–1
  bone mineralization and 32

collagen (*contd*)
  type I 30, 32, *32*
collagen-derived peptides, crosslinked 38–9
Colles' fracture 7
  see also forearm fractures, distal
computed tomography, quantitative (QCT) 4, *5*
contingent valuation 83
Cooper, Sir Astley 1
coronary heart disease (CHD) 60, 61
corticosteroids (glucocorticoids) 33, 38
  avoidance 70
  fracture risk 49, *50*
  in fracture risk assessment 51
cost-benefit analysis 83
cost effectiveness
  fracture prevention treatments 85–98
  targeting treatments 98–9
cost-effectiveness acceptability curves (CEAC) 84, *85*
cost-effectiveness analysis 82
  addressing uncertainty 84
  validity of results 97–8
costs
  in economic evaluations 82
  fracture-related 21–3, *22*
cost-utility analysis 82–3
cytokines 35–6

definition of osteoporosis 2–3
  BMD perspective 3–6
  fracture perspective 3, 6
  WHO 2–3, *4*, 44
diagnosis of osteoporosis 43, 44
  WHO criteria 2–3, *4*
diet *see* nutrition
1,25-dihydroxycholecalciferol (1,25–(OH)$_2$D$_3$) 37
disability, fracture-related 18–20, *20*
dual X-ray absorptiometry (DXA or DEXA) 4, *5, 6*

economics 81–102, 115–16
  addressing uncertainty 84
  evaluation methods 81–3
  fracture prevention treatments 85–97
  targeting treatments 98–9
  validity of evaluations 97–8
epidemiology 13–26
ergocalciferol 37
estrogen 33, 38
  agonists and antagonists 60–1
  replacement therapy *see* hormone replacement
    therapy
ethnic differences
  fracture rates 16, 17–18
  osteoporosis prevalence *14*, 14–15
etidronate
  cost effectiveness *90, 91*
  efficacy 64, 88
European Foundation for Osteoporosis and Bone
  Disease (EFFO) 103, *107, 108*

European Society of Musculoskeletal Radiology 8
exercise 69, 104–5

falls 9–10, 17, 106
  prevention 69, 70, 106
  risk factors 48–9, 106
femoral neck fractures *see* hip fractures
FIT studies *62, 63, 64*
fluoride 67
forearm fractures, distal 7
  frequency *16,* 17–18
  lifetime risk 18
  morbidity 19–20, *20*
  mortality 21
  prior *50*
  risk assessment 45, *45*
fracture(s) 6–10
  burden 9–10
  costs 21–3
  defining osteoporosis 3, 6
  definition 6–8
  determinants of risk 9
  economic aspects 81–102
  family history 99
  frequency 16–18
  historical perspectives 1–2
  morbidity 18–20, *19, 20*
  mortality 20–1, *21*
  orthopedic management 69–70
  prevention strategies *see* prevention strategies
  prior 49, *50,* 51, 98–9
  risk factors *see* risk factors
  treatment options 71
  see also specific fracture sites
FRACTURE Index *112,* 112–13, *113*
fracture risk
  age-specific estimates *115*
  assessment *see* risk assessment
  BMD and 109
  choice of therapy and 70–1
  lifetime 9, 18, 46
  pharmacological reduction *57,* 59, 61, 64–6
  relative *vs* absolute 46, 114–16
  see also high-risk patients
frequency
  fractures 16–18
  osteoporosis 13–15, 44, *45*
functional impairment, fracture-related 18–19, *20*

gamble, standard 83
gender differences *see* sex differences
genetic factors, bone mass 33
geographic variations, fracture rates 16, 17–18
glucocorticoids *see* corticosteroids
growth hormone (GH)
  effects on bone 33, 38
  therapy 68

Haversian systems 29
HERS study 60, 87
high-risk patients
    identifying 2–3, 43–55
    targeting treatment to 98–9
hip fractures
    classification 7, 7
    costs 22, 22–3
    definition 7
    economics of prevention 89
    frequency 16, 16
    historical perspectives 1
    lifetime risk 18
    morbidity 18–19, 20
    mortality 20–1, 21
    orthopedic management 69
    pharmacological prevention 63, 65, 67, 88
    physical prevention 70
    prior 50
    risk assessment 45, 45–6, 47, 47, 51, 51
    risk scoring 110, 111, 111–13, 113
hip protectors 70, 106
hormone replacement therapy (HRT) 59–60
    cost effectiveness 85–7, 88, 99
    effectiveness 59, 86, 86
    indications 71
    vs other treatments 73
hydroxyapatite 32
hydroxyproline, urinary total 38–9
25-hydroxyvitamin D (25(OH)D) 37
hypercalcemia 37, 38

ibandronate 66
incidence of fractures 16, 16, 17–18
inositol triphosphate 36
International Osteoporosis Foundation (IOF) 8, 44,
    46, 72
ipriflavone 68

marble bone disease 33
menatetrenone 68
menopause, early or surgical 99
Million Women Study 60, 61
morbidity, fracture-related 18–20, 19, 20
MORE (Multiple Outcomes of Raloxifene
    Evaluation) study 61, 62, 63
mortality, fracture-related 20–1, 21

National Health and Nutrition Examination Survey
    (NHANES) 14, 15
National Osteoporosis Foundation (NOF) 103,
    106–8, 107
number needed to treat (NNT) 114–15
nutrition 33, 68–9, 104

orthopedic management, osteoporotic fractures
    69–70
osteoblasts 29, 30, 33
    biochemical measures of activity 38–9
osteocalcin 38, 39

osteoclast-activating factors (OAFs) 36
osteoclasts 33, 34
osteocytes 30, 34
osteogenesis imperfecta 32
osteomalacia 2, 32
osteopenia
    definition 4
    treatment 71
osteopetrosis 33
osteoporosis
    definitions 2–3, 4, 44
    severe (established) 4, 44
Osteoporosis Society of Canada (OSC) 103, 107,
    108–9

pamidronate 65–6
parathyroid hormone (PTH) 33, 37
    mechanism of action 73
    recombinant human 1–34 fragment
        (rhPTH(1–34)) 62, 63, 66–7
    therapy 66–7, 71, 73
parathyroid hormone-related protein (PTHrP) 38
pathophysiology of osteoporosis 2, 27–41
peak bone mass 27, 28
pharmacological therapy 57, 58–68
    indications 108–9, 116
    selection of agents 70–1
    see also specific agents
phosphate balance 36–8
physical activity 69, 104–5
postmenopausal osteoporosis
    frequency 14, 44, 45
    historical perspectives 1–2
    treatment 57–80
postmenopausal women
    loss of bone mass 28
    vertebral fractures 17
prevalence, osteoporosis 13–14
prevention strategies 103–18
    BMD-based 109
    combined risk factors (risk scores) 109–14
    relative risk, absolute risk and risk difference
        114–16
    risk factor-based 103–9
    see also treatment
progestins 59–60
PROOF study 62, 63, 66
proteins, non-collagen bone 31
proteoglycans 31
PTH see parathyroid hormone

quality adjusted life years (QALYs) 81, 82–3
quality of life, impact of fractures 19, 20
quantitative computed tomography (QCT) 4, 5
quantitative ultrasound (QUS) 4, 5, 6

racial differences see ethnic differences
radiographic absorptiometry 5
radiography, plain 3, 8

STEPPING HILL HOSPITAL
LIBRARY
PINEWOOD

raloxifene 60–1
    efficacy 61, *62, 63*
    indications 71
    vs other treatments 72, 73
relative risk 46, 114–16, *115*
rickets 32, 37
risedronate
    cost effectiveness 84, *85,* 88, *91*
    efficacy *62, 63,* 65
    vs other treatments 73
risk
    absolute 46, 114–16, *115*
    fracture *see* fracture risk
    relative 46, 114–16, *115*
risk assessment 2–3, 43–4, 45–52
    age and BMD *47,* 47–8, *48*
    biochemical markers 50
    other risk factors 48–9, *49*
    risk factor integration 48–9, *49*
risk difference 114–16
risk factors 43, 103–8, *107*
    behavioral and environmental 104–6
    BMD determination and 106–8
    integration 48–9, *49,* 109–14
    intrinsic 106–8
    targeting treatment and 98–9
risk scoring systems 109–14, *110, 112*
risk stratification 43–55
Royal College of Physicians of Great Britain (RCP)
    103, *107,* 108
RUTH study 61

selective estrogen receptor modulators (SERMs) 60–1
sensitivity analysis 84, 98
sex differences
    age-related loss of bone mass 28, *28*
    fracture frequency 16, *16,* 17
    fracture-related mortality 20–1, *21*
    lifetime fracture risk 18
    osteoporosis frequency 15
sex hormones 38
single X-ray absorptiometry (SXA) 4, *5*
Smith's fracture 7
smoking, cigarette 99, 105
SOF *see* Study of Osteoporotic Fractures
spine fractures *see* vertebral fractures
statins 68
stress, mechanical 33
strontium ranelate 68
Study of Osteoporotic Fractures (SOF or SOFt) 98,
    99, 109, *112,* 112–13

tamoxifen 60
testosterone 27, 33
thiazide diuretics 68
thyroxine 38
tibolone 61
tiludronate 65
time trade off methods 83

transforming growth factor-β (TGF-β) proteins 32
trauma, causing fractures 9–10
treatment 57–80
    BMD thresholds 43–4, 71, 108–9, 116
    choice of agent 70–1
    cost effectiveness 85–97
    high-risk patients without fractures 71
    indications 73, 108–9, 116
    monitoring 72
    nonpharmacologic 68–70
    patients with fractures 71
    pharmacological *57,* 58–68
    risk stratification 52
    targeting 98–9
    see also prevention strategies
T-score
    diagnostic use 4, 6, 44
    fracture risk assessment *45,* 45–8, *47, 48*
    intervention thresholds 43–4, 71, 108–9, 116

ultrasound, quantitative (QUS) 4, *5,* 6
uncertainty, in economic evaluations 84
utilities 82–3

vertebral fractures 8
    definition 8
    frequency *16,* 17
    historical perspectives 2
    lifetime risk 18
    morbidity 19, *20*
    mortality rates 21
    nonpharmacologic interventions 69
    orthopedic management 69–70
    pharmacological prevention *57,* 61, *62,* 64, 65,
        66–7
    prior *49, 50,* 99
    risk assessment *45,* 46, 47–8, *48*
    treatment options 71
VERT-MN study *62, 63*
VERT-US study *62, 63*
vitamin D 37
    analogs 67
    cost effectiveness 92–7, *93–6,* 98, 100
    dietary intake 69, 104
    supplements 58–9
vitamin D receptors 37
vitamin K 67–8

willingness to pay 83
Wolff's law 33
Women's Health Initiative (WHI) study 59, 60, 86, 87
World Health Organization (WHO)
    definition of osteoporosis 2–3, *4,* 44
    fracture risk assessment 46
wrist fractures *see* forearm fractures, distal

X-ray absorptiometry 4, *5*

zoledronate 66
Z-score 4

£40.00.